TAKE 5

A Transformative Diet Lifestyle in the Era of the Coronavirus

By Kenneth Derow, MBA

Consumer Behavior Expert

First Edition

Copyright 2020, Salvage Writes Media

978-1-7335757-4-4

Dedication

This book is dedicated to my wife. Without her unwavering and loving support over the past fifty years, and, particularly over the past 8 years during which I have labored on this project, it would truly never have been undertaken or completed. Thank you Carol for your love, support and encouragement.

Acknowledgements

There are many people who I could rightfully acknowledge for helping me along over this eight-year journey. First, and foremost, among them is my family. My daughter, Jennifer Salvage and my son-in-law Jeff Salvage. Their tireless efforts and support of my project, not to mention acting as a sounding board for my ideas, as editors and as my muse, was invaluable. Thank you so much, Jen and Jeff.

There were also numerous professionals, medical and scientific advisers I need to acknowledge as well. For much of the eight years during which I researched, developed and wrote this book, I was collaborating with Harvard Med/Mass General Hospital, neuroscientist, Dr. Rudy Tanzi. His comments, his encouragement and at times, his prodding was instrumental in getting the ideas in this book better articulated and well-grounded in brain science and psychology. Over the years, our relationship has blossomed into a friendship. Thank you Rudy!

Two other people, both physicians and nutrition/obesity experts who came into my life not too long ago, have also helped me immensely. Dr. Meagan Grega, a highly regarded nutrition/obesity and lifestyle expert, gave me great advice and commentary that I have incorporated into the book. And, Yale University's Dr. David Katz, an eminent nutrition/obesity educator and researcher, was an inspiration to me and made me work harder and better to improve the book's core ideas. Thank you Meagan and David!

Table of Contents

Foreword

There is no debate regarding the epidemic of obesity and chronic disease in our society. It has become atypical for adults to maintain their weight in a healthy range throughout their lifetime. Additionally, Americans take more prescription medications than do citizens of any other country in the world. If you are a middle-age adult in this country with a BMI (Body Mass Index) under 25 and do not take medication for a chronic disease, you are an anomaly. We are experiencing an epidemic of poor health, decreased energy and lack of vitality.

How did this happen? Cardiovascular disease is our number one killer, with one American dying approximately every 40 seconds from this largely preventable and reversible disease. Diabetes is also rising at an alarming rate throughout our population, with the CDC now predicting that 2 out of 5 Americans will develop diabetes during their lifetime. In contrast, in 1960 the diabetes rate in America was approximately 1% of the population. What changed? We know that it cannot be due to genetic shifts over such a short time span. It must be related to environmental factors that shape our lifestyle choices; resulting in alterations in what and how much we eat, how often we move, how well we sleep, how we handle stress, how connected we are to a social support system and whether we possess a strong sense of purpose.

A lot has changed over the past six decades in the way we live our lives. Some of these changes have been extremely positive, such as improved gender and racial equality and increased access to information and educational resources through rapidly expanding internet connectivity. Unfortunately, we also changed in ways that resulted in appalling increases in chronic disease rates, often called diseases of affluence or non-communicable diseases, such as heart disease, cancer, diabetes, hypertension, high cholesterol and Alzheimer's disease. Obesity increases the risk of developing all of these conditions, and, in itself, presents a major risk to our health.

We created a society where health-promoting habits are often discouraged; either by the physical environment of the communities where we live, the frenetic pace of our daily schedules or the social norms surrounding us via friends, family and co-workers. Highly-processed convenience foods that provide temporary pleasure while eating them, but are very calorie-dense and nutrient-light, are abundantly available and jeopardize our longevity and vitality. Not only are these ultra-processed foods easily accessible, the number of tempting varieties also exploded. From the donuts and muffins prominently displayed in most work-site break rooms to the goodie bags sent home from birthday parties and school or sporting events and the veritable cornucopia of fast-food options available on even a short drive through the majority of our neighborhoods, we are surrounded by cheap, convenient, very high-calorie, but nutritionally-empty foods. These are foods that are virtually, addictively palatable and thereby very difficult to resist.

How can we combat these pervasive influences and achieve not only a long lifespan, but a long healthspan; which means aging with vitality and purpose, able to engage with our families, friends and favorite activities? One of the most powerful tools we can use is to arrange our personal environment to support the habits proven to be associated with good health. Mindfulness is at the very core of the Whole Brain Diet Lifestyle and the Take 5 technique. Utilizing mindfulness-based approaches such as Take 5 is a highly effective strategy to manage our responses to food and to lower our frustration and stress in a way that leads to lasting weight loss and the ability to achieve our goals for longevity, vigor and happiness. It is a simple tool that, when practiced regularly, can re-wire our habitual responses to common situations and change our life.

It may seem that cravings and distracted, mindless eating are an inescapable part of the frenetic pace of modern life, as unavoidable as death and taxes; but this distressing version of reality does not need to be so. However, it is true that we are surrounded by highly-processed, hyper-palatable but nutritionally-deficient food options which require intention and awareness to navigate and avoid. Intention and awareness have never been more urgent than now, in the era of the Coronavirus 19, when so many of us are confined to our homes for an extended period of time, managing meals for multiple family members while dealing with significantly increased levels of stress. Fortunately, the Take 5 technique is an excellent tool to refocus and support conscious decisions regarding food choices. Take 5 allows us to break the momentum of the powerful physical-emotional craving impulses that drive us to eat, often in a semi-automatic, non-thinking manner.

A 2019 research study highlighted the difficulty of self-regulation and the disruption of internal satiety signals when eating a highly processed, typical American diet. Adults enrolled in the study were offered ultra-processed diets for 14 days and unprocessed, whole food diets for a separate 14 days in a random order. The two study diets were matched for presented calories, sugar, fat, fiber and macronutrient content. Study subjects were allowed to eat as much, or as little, of the food presented during each 14 day period as they desired. The results provide an insightful window into the cause of expanding waistlines of many Americans today. During the ultra-processed segment of the dietary intervention study, subjects consumed approximately 500 calories more per day than the exact same participants consumed when they were offered the unprocessed diet. As a result, the study subjects gained weight during the ultra-processed dietary portion of the study and lost weight during the unprocessed dietary phase, without any outside restrictions on their eating habits.

How can we combat the ubiquitous, unhealthful food choices that surround us, like ultra-processed foods? The mindfulness techniques outlined in the Take 5 approach provide a roadmap for noticing and then diffusing the cravings we may experience as we take steps to implement a healthier lifestyle. Master Buddhist teacher Thich Nhat Hanh has stated "When we take a moment to sit and breathe before we eat, we can get in touch with the real hunger in our body. We can discover if we're eating because we're hungry or if we're eating because it's the time to eat and the food is there." Similarly, one of the foundational pillars of the Okinawan Blue Zone, which boasts some of the longest lived inhabitants in the world, is the concept of Hara Hachi Bu, which roughly translates to "Eat until you are 80% full." Utilizing the "punctuated eating" process described in Take 5, the heart of the Whole Brain Diet Lifestyle, provides an innovative way to operationalize the concepts of purposefully savoring your food and ending your meal before you become uncomfortable due to overeating.

Another important approach involves configuring your environment to minimize exposure to undesirable food choices or cues that may trigger cravings. Creating your surroundings so that the default choice is the optimal choice is a powerful way to successfully transition to more nourishing and healthful habits. Equally as important is the active participation of your friends and family members. Social nudges – the norms and routines that are practiced by those around us – are a formidable influence on our own behavior. By enlisting the assistance of your support system, as strongly advocated as part of the Whole Brain Diet Lifestyle, you increase your own likelihood of making substantial lifestyle changes, as well as helping to improve the health and vitality of the people most important to you. The Take 5 technique provides actionable steps to minimize your exposure to unhealthy cravings and to consciously diffuse any cravings that occur, while still allowing you to savor delicious, satisfying food.

The approach described in the Whole Brain Diet Lifestyle, powered by the Take 5 technique, can help you reach your goals, whether that goal is to lose weight, reverse chronic disease or maintain your health and vigor. By transforming your lifestyle, you fundamentally change your life. Try it and see where Take 5 can take you!

Meagan L. Grega, MD, FACLM
Co-Founder, Chief Medical Officer Kellyn Foundation
Board Certified in Family Medicine and Lifestyle Medicine
www.kellyn.org

Prologue
The invisible hand of evolutionary forces forged our instincts and drives much of our behavior.

A War Between Fat and Thin
A battle is raging across households throughout this country, a battle that will literally determine the long-run health of American families. It is the battle between fat and thin, and fat is clearly winning the war. Over 70% of adults in this country are overweight, and approximately 40% are considered obese.[1] America is in the midst of several widely acknowledged epidemics, including an increasing number of people who are obese, diabetic or have heart disease, all largely preventable conditions.[2] This is one important reason why there are a huge number of diet books published each year. The demand for healthy solutions is extremely large, but very poorly satisfied.

Traditional books giving diet advice, plans and menus simply do not work in the long-run. It is well documented that 95% of people who lose a significant amount of weight regain it all, and even more, over the following two years after dieting.[3] It is true that those who closely adhere to almost any of these popular diets, whether very low-carb or low-fat, high-protein or some other even more esoteric and bizarre plan, lose weight. If you follow any diet you consume fewer calories and therefore lose weight. It is not hard to understand why these plans typically never provide evidence on maintaining that weight loss over time, as almost all dieters fail to do this successfully.

My own weight challenge was a constant struggle. My weight ballooned to over two hundred pounds. It was not a rapid rise, but a slow seemingly inexorable year-to-year increase that seemed to stealthily creep up and overtake me. Feeling uncomfortable and unwell at that weight, I entered a long process of trying and ultimately rejecting various diets. I tried traditional diets, and even tried some bizarre fad diets. They worked for a while to produce a weight loss, but none produced a weight loss that lasted. I was frustrated, but resolved to find a way of producing a more permanent weight loss.

With this as motivation, I read everything I could find on diets, dieting and the psychology of eating and overeating. I studied the role of cravings on our behavior. I read the latest findings in brain science and human behavior and how it might relate to developing, a healthful diet lifestyle that worked. Finally, it all came together, not in a *Eureka Moment*, but I slowly realized that I had a radical paradigm shift that could help myself to lose weight and keep it off. This was the genesis for creating the Whole Brain Diet Lifestyle.

Starting at around two hundred pounds, I ultimately lost a total of forty pounds over eighteen months and maintained that loss for over six years. My weight loss was not rapid, but it was steady and consistent (one key to why the Whole Brain Diet Lifestyle plan works). This book is the culmination of eight years of research, experimentation and deep contemplative thinking. It encapsulates much of what I've learned about how to combat obesity in a manner that is both healthy and lasting.

The Whole Brain Diet Lifestyle plan is not a diet; it is a highly detailed and comprehensive lifestyle plan that demonstrates how to dramatically transform your relationship to eating and snacking, along many complementary dimensions. I show specifically how you can use your brain to master your behavior and how to create a psychological, social, and physical environment that strongly nudges you in a more healthful direction. Your environment exerts a powerful and under-appreciated influence on your behavior.

At its heart, the Whole Brain Diet Lifestyle is based on the premise that, metaphorically speaking, all humans have a *Fat* brain housed in the ancient reptilian part of their brain and a *Skinny* brain housed in the newest part of the brain, the neocortex. This is a critically important point, but remember, it is simply a metaphorical convenience. The Whole Brain Diet Lifestyle refers to a set of behaviors that appeal to your need and desire to live a healthful lifestyle and to weigh less. It does not refer to an aspiration to literally become "skinny."

This is an important distinction. The Whole Brain Diet Lifestyle is about learning to change how, when and what you eat and how to transform your relationship with food. That is, how to live a healthier life. If you follow the plan, one key byproduct is weight loss, but is only one of the ways the plan makes you healthier and improves your overall well-being. Becoming skinny is not an objective of the Whole Brain Diet Lifestyle and is not indicative of living a truly healthy life!

Imperative Evolutionary Instincts

Instincts bred into your DNA by millions of years of evolutionary history are still imprinted on your brain today and greatly affect your behavior in fundamental ways. The basic incompatibility between these ancient drives and our modern world cause you to act in ways that actually counter the reasons these instincts initially developed.

Your brain presents you with a conundrum I call the *Fat* brain – *Skinny* brain dichotomy, and the name adopted for the diet lifestyle plan detailed in this book is the Whole Brain Diet Lifestyle. A million years of evolutionary instincts drive us, even compel us, to eat whenever and whatever is available in large quantities. This drive is even stronger for high-sugar, high-simple-carb, high-calorie foods. These foods are commonly referred to as junk foods and make up a large proportion of ultra-processed foods.

The brain's natural state is to strive to be fat, to provide a safe and comfortable margin of fat to sustain us through times when food energy sources are scarce or non-existent. This was true throughout most of the history of Homo sapiens and our primate ancestors when starvation was an operative challenge. The most basic behavioral imperative embedded in our DNA is for self-preservation. This imprint in the most primal and ancient part of our brain is incredibly powerful.

In the newest part of the brain, the neocortex, we have a conscious self-awareness and desire to be thin for a multitude of psychosocial and health reasons. One critical reason is that in many cultures being thin is advantageous to attracting a sexual partner and mate. Along with self-preservation, the instinct to pass on our genes through our offspring is an extremely powerful force, which helps to drive our desire to be thin and more attractive others.

Within in each of us there is this ongoing conflict, a conundrum, between our *Fat* brain and our *Skinny* brain. To effectively deal with this conflict, we must first be aware of it, and then have strategies, tools and techniques to manage it.

Your *Skinny* brain needs to be alert, focused and vigilant to override the omnipresent *Fat* brain, or it will lose the battle to control your behavior. Your ancient subconscious brain wants to be fat. Your newer conscious brain wants to be thin. How can you resolve this dilemma? That is the ultimate purpose of this book, using a combination of brain science, psychology and common sense.

The *Fat* brain – *Skinny* brain dichotomy is supported in the paradigm-shifting work of Nobel Prize winner Daniel Kahneman. In his book *Thinking Fast and Slow*,[4] he describes two modes or styles of thinking, one fast and unconscious (he termed it System 1), one slow and deliberate (System 2). Your *Fat* brain (working fast and unconsciously) and your *Skinny* brain (working slow and deliberately) parallel the essential premise of Kahneman's theory. One of the core goals of the Whole Brain Diet Lifestyle brain plan is to help shift your thinking and behavioral responses away from a subconscious mode into a conscious state where your *Skinny* brain is in control. In this way, following the dictates of your *Skinny* brain becomes more natural and less subject to the impulsive, high-sugar, high-calorie cravings that we all experience. When this occurs, real dietary lifestyle transformation is possible and likely.

I describe in detail a tool to help you rapidly and easily shift your thinking and your responses from a virtually automatic and unconscious System 1 mode, to a more deliberate and conscious System 2. I call this tool ***Take 5***. The Take 5 tool is central to the Whole Brain Diet Lifestyle plan as it encapsulates and operationalizes the principle of mindfulness on which the entire lifestyle is based and allows you to immediately disarm a craving impulse.

Quieting Evolutionary Instincts

This book clearly and specifically shows you how you can quiet a million years of evolutionary instincts that drive overeating and obesity. You will learn how to quiet the extraneous thoughts that bubble up from your subconscious, which otherwise create a craving to eat unhealthfully, snack inappropriately or overeat. The tools and techniques allow you to Stop, Think, Observe and Process (i.e., to STOP) a choice and detach from a feeling without acting upon it. By aligning your higher-level conscious intentions with your subconscious emotional brain to command your attention, you silence cravings and drive your behavior in a more healthful manner. The Take 5 technique is central to achieving this objective.

Establishing Habitual Behaviors

To resolve the ever-present *Fat* brain – *Skinny* brain conundrum, you must learn how to establish new habits to carry you through to a permanently changed behavioral state. Establishing and relying on positive habits allows you to bypass your sole reliance on your willpower, which is embedded in your higher-level conscious brain, and to utilize the incredible power of your subconscious emotional brain. When these two parts of your brain are aligned supporting a common goal, there is little that you cannot accomplish.

The key to achieving new habits is to learn how to rewire the neural network in your brain. A rewired brain brings you to a world in which you naturally and automatically choose a healthy, nutritious diet and where your high-sugar, high-calorie cravings are significantly diminished. And when you do experience an emotional impulse to eat unhealthfully, you activate new automatic responses, like Take 5, that become habitual and allow you to counter and defuse the impulse.

You can use your conscious intentions to initiate the process of change, but intent and willpower alone is usually not enough. Willpower is too readily depleted to carry you through to long-term behavioral change. There is a period of maximum vulnerability when you are trying to achieve transformational change in your behavior. This is the transitional time between one's initial intention to change and the establishment of new routines and habits. This phase is when most people fall prey to insufficient willpower and resolve to stay the course. I explain how to overcome this natural impediment and take deliberate actions to maximize the mental energy needed to supercharge your willpower and build as well as sustain your self-control.

Your brain resists change as it naturally favors constancy and familiarity. But I show you how to power through this resistance and overcome the natural inertia your brain creates, by increasing the growth and connectivity of the neural networks in your brain. This is how new habits are formed and established. Once new healthier routines are instilled, the brain acts to preserve them, as it once did for the less healthy habits that you had. Ultimately, true long-term transformational behavioral change can become a reality.

Who Will Benefit from a Whole Brain Diet Lifestyle?

The scientific evidence and common sense are abundantly clear: while it can be difficult to maintain your existing weight, it is even harder to lose weight and keep it off. This book is written not only for those who are currently obese or overweight, but also many others who are struggling to maintain their weight, or simply fear that their weight will surreptitiously and slowly creep up over time. Even more important, this book is designed for anyone who desires a healthier lifestyle. Of course, this includes almost all American adults and a high percentage of adults throughout the Western world—that's why this book is right for you!

One important reason that this book is appropriate for so many people is that the Whole Brain Diet Lifestyle plan has many facets, many elements and is thereby highly robust and highly flexible. One advantage of this plan is that unlike most other traditional diet programs or diet lifestyles, it is not highly prescriptive nor highly restrictive. In most old-fashioned diets, especially the fad ones, you must adhere to every aspect of the plan or it fails. With the Whole Brain Diet Lifestyle plan, you have the power to customize it to meet your personal needs.

The Whole Brain Diet Lifestyle plan is analogous to a huge Chinese restaurant menu. Except, instead of having a choice of one from Column A and one from Column B, you can choose any number of items you want from many columns. Based on how appetizing the strategy or tactic is to you and how well you feel you can incorporate it into your life for the long-term determines which items you want to select. The plan gives you the power to experiment. There is no single best combination of elements that is right for everyone.

Start with those elements that make sense to you, try them and see how they work. Keep those that seem to help; jettison those that do not. If you are progressing acceptably toward your goal of dietary behavioral lifestyle transformation and weight loss, continue as is. If not, go back and reconfigure your personal plan and try again. You have options; you have choices; the Whole Brain Diet Lifestyle puts the power in your hands.

Serendipitously, the highly robust and multifaceted nature of the Whole Brain Diet Lifestyle has another benefit derived from the freedom of choice that it offers. This freedom requires you to be actively involved in the process of configuring the exact array of tactics and tools you plan to use to achieve your lifestyle goals. This involvement makes your buy-in to the plan much more likely and generates greater engagement on your part. More engagement means that you are more likely to stick with it long enough for new routines to become habitual. Good, positive habits are the key to your achieving your diet lifestyle goals.

A Diet Lifestyle in the Era of Coronavirus

The Whole Brain Diet Lifestyle plan, powered by the Take 5 technique, is uniquely well-suited to be the lifestyle of choice in the era of the Coronavirus. Take 5 works on two different levels.

First and foremost, in the new era of extended self-isolation in our homes, for so many of us, our access to food and snacks, especially ultra-processed foods and junk foods, has gone from being metaphorically 24/7, to literally 24/7. With perpetual accessibility, fueled by high stress and high anxiety, it has never been more difficult to resist the temptation to eat, and overeat, unhealthful foods, fostering weight gain, and the onset of obesity.

The Take 5 technique is the perfect antidote to ameliorate the physical-emotional cravings driving us to eat/overeat unhealthful foods, by providing a brief buffer period to allow these craving impulses to dissipate and also by helping us to mitigate the stress of confinement and our very understandable virus-related fears. This diet lifestyle also works to deter unhealthful snacking by constructing psychological, social and physical barriers to significantly reduce our ready accessibility to food, and especially to junk foods. The Take 5 tool and the comprehensive Whole Brain Diet Lifestyle plan, both work to help us eat more healthful foods and overeat less.

On a second level, the Whole Brain Diet Lifestyle, powered by Take 5, aids those who follow the plan to fight the Coronavirus, by helping us to lose weight, reduce stress and eat/overeat less ultra-processed/junk foods. Weight gain and obesity-driven consumption of junk foods are known to depress and weaken our immune system functioning. Based on data from abroad and from the CDC, after "old age," the factor that is most highly correlated with getting Covid-19, requiring hospitalization and for some, subsequent death, is obesity. A strong well-functioning immune system may mitigate some of this risk. Overall, this diet lifestyle helps one to lose weight, deter the onset of obesity, reduce inflammation and strengthen the immune system, making it the ideal choice in these perilous times.

WEIGHTLESS – The Ultimate State of Being

The final and ultimate stage of the Whole Brain Diet Lifestyle is to enter a state where you become what I call weightless. Being weightless is a metaphor for a state of being, of the mind and body, which we can all achieve. It is a state where our typical, frequent preoccupation with food, diets and weight is replaced by a new equilibrium. This gives balance to your life, where you eat and live healthfully as your natural default mode. Being weightless becomes a natural and automatic way of life, a philosophy for living. Your *Skinny* brain becomes much more active as its intent now resides in both your conscious and subconscious parts of your brain, giving it the power to better counter your *Fat* brain's natural instinct to eat and overeat.

Using the Whole Brain Diet Lifestyle is the path to achieving this weightless state of being, where you have internalized and made habitual a mindful awareness that provides a brief buffer moment in which your deliberate, conscious intent to align with and follow your *Skinny* brain happens automatically. When you reach a true state of weightlessness, the ever-present internal tension and conflicting demands of your *Fat* brain and your *Skinny* brain impulses disappear, and your mind and your body are at peace, not in a state of constant tension.

Not to become too metaphysical or sound too new-agey, but achieving a state of weightlessness is a higher order of consciousness than most of us typically realize. You become more in tune with your body, your mind and your spirit. They all work together toward a more healthful lifestyle. Being weightless is a pursuit with no end, no final finish line. The intrinsic rewards this pursuit gives to your body and mind are sustainable for a lifetime and continues to motivate you ever more toward a better life and a higher state of well-being.

Of course, to achieve this state requires commitment and sustained effort to reach, but it is doable. The great multiplicity of strategies, tactics and tools the Whole Brain Diet Lifestyle plan offers allows you to configure a specific combination of elements that work for you. While you might choose to rely solely on the Take 5 technique to reach your desired weight, and an improved overall well-being, for those who need or want it, the Whole Brain Diet Lifestyle plan offers you so much more. Finish reading *TAKE 5*, select the parts of the plan you find appealing and workable for you and you will be on a path whose end point is a natural progression into a weightless state of being.

Becoming weightless is a choice. Your brain gives you the power and if you want it to happen, you can definitely make it so. As Rudy Tanzi describes in *Super Brain* (co-authored with Deepak Chopra), you can be the user of your brain, or let it use you. When you exercise control and dominance over your impulses by using the Whole Brain Diet Lifestyle, you can enter a weightless state and immeasurably improve your health and well-being.

You might ask whether achieving a weightless state of being can be a reality for you, or is it merely an aspirational state to strive for? Today, those that know me as a healthy, slim individual would never believe I once was disturbingly obese, completely out of shape and an eating machine. For most of my adult life I indulged my taste and desire to consume volumes of highly palatable foods, over those my brain told me were actually much more healthful. The immediate reward was often replaced with a sense of dread over guilty feelings for indulging my *Fat* brain and often the physical discomfort from stuffing myself to the point where I felt the need to throw up; but I did it anyway. My kids arrived at the dinner table ready to race to consume their meals for fear the "Hoover vac" would steal unattended morsels from their plates before they could finish their meals. Today, that person is a complete stranger to me.

A few years ago, after incorporating the Whole Brain Diet Lifestyle into my daily routine, I entered a state of weightlessness. When I was deciding what to have for lunch and I spontaneously chose to have a plate of raw, fresh vegetables (with a small serving of low calorie dressing). I had not ever done this before. I realized that far from dreading eating this meal or regretting a hasty choice, I was actually looking forward to it. I ate it, enjoyed it and felt good about my choice afterward.

Suddenly, I had two realizations, an epiphany of sorts. First, I knew I would choose and enjoy this veggie smorgasbord many more times in the future. Secondly, I knew that I was now weightless. The desire for sugary, high-calorie foods wasn't eliminated entirely, nor was all inappropriate snacking and overeating eliminated, but such behaviors were minimized. A state where the constant confrontation and tension between my *Fat* brain and my *Skinny* brain was not one hundred percent gone, but was significantly reduced. A state where, when a craving for a high-sugar, high-calorie food did emerge, it now held less urgency and dissipated more quickly.

I knew in my heart and in my gut that becoming seriously overweight was never going to be a troubling concern for me ever again. The "war" between my *Fat* brain and my *Skinny* brain was waged and my *Skinny* brain emerged victorious. I followed elements of the Whole Brain Diet Lifestyle closely to lose my initial weight. Now that I have entered into a weightless state of being, keeping the weight off requires much less vigilance and much less ongoing effort. The war between fat and thin is over for me.

Becoming weightless can be a real state of being and this is how I know that you too can become weightless. It does not happen immediately, nor overnight, but with persistence and the creation of new positive habits you develop by following the Whole Brain Diet Lifestyle, it can happen.

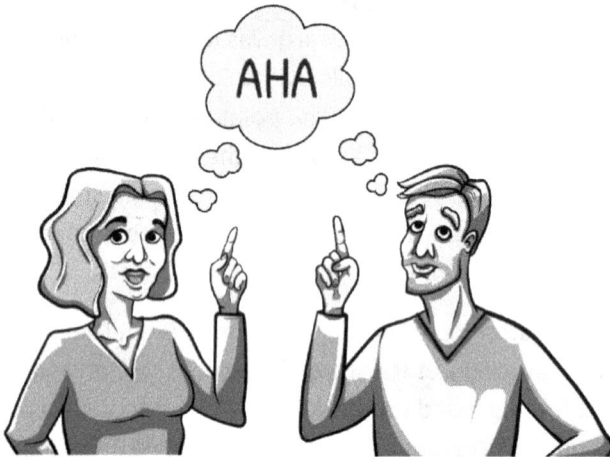

- Of course, your brain is not literally divided into a *Fat* brain and a *Skinny* brain. Both desires reside simultaneously in different parts of your brain, creating a dynamic of constant tension between the two. This book teaches you how to quiet the ever-present impulses from your *Fat* brain while enhancing and strengthening the messages your *Skinny* brain is sending to you.
- Primal instincts are real and powerful, but, if you persevere, you can consciously use your brain to redirect and to counter them. This book is all about how to accomplish this.

Introduction

Over the course of our long evolutionary history, obesity was virtually unknown, starvation was the real operative challenge and our brains adapted to this environment with significant real-world consequences.

Primal Behavioral Imperatives

Virtually all of the behavior of living organisms, including humans, flows from and is driven by two interconnected forces that are embedded in our DNA and manifested in our instincts. The instinctive drives are the dual behavioral imperatives of self-preservation and replicating our DNA via our offspring.[1] These drives ensure our preservation as individuals and as a species. As Richard Brodie says in his book *Virus of the Mind,* from our DNA's point of view, having copies of it is "our whole point for existing."[2]

Because our instincts are not readily accessible to our conscious mind, we very significantly discount and underestimate their impact on our decision-making and our behavior. The conscious mind always seeks a rationale to explain and justify our behavior, but we seldom have the level of self-awareness and knowledge necessary to discern the real drivers. When you dive deep into what drives your motivations, you find that taking actions to preserve one's self, seek sex or care for our partner and offspring are often at the core.

At one level or another, almost all of our behavior via our deep subconscious is influenced and activated by these very fundamental and primal forces. Many behaviors that were critical for our survival and DNA replication developed early in our evolutionary history to sustain and promote preservation of the species. Some of them are inappropriate or inconsistent in today's world, and even run counter to the original purpose that caused these instincts to be programmed into our DNA.[4]

Early Homo sapiens: An Era of Food Scarcity

To survive in the pre-human or early hominid era required great endurance and extreme physical exertion to hunt or gather very scarce, inaccessible, and/or dangerous food sources. This was highly energy-depleting, i.e., it burned a lot of calories. Before the agricultural revolution when crops were planted, man had to track and kill their prey, or gather food from sometimes remote, sparse, natural food sources. Overabundance of food was never an issue or a problem. If people were lucky enough for a major kill to feed themselves and/or their clan, it all had to be consumed quickly, as food preservation was still unknown. In the early days of humanity, one ate whenever, wherever, and whatever one could, as the timing of the next kill, or next meal was uncertain.[5]

Our brain adapted to an era of food scarcity and an uncertain and unknown accessibility to food energy sources that required great physical exertion to provide sustenance. When food was available, gorging oneself favored survival, and obesity was unknown. There was no junk food, fast food, refrigeration, and no idle, mindless snacking. Hominids (pre-Homo sapiens) and humans naturally learned to eat whenever food was available and to consume as large a quantity as was possible. For virtually all of mankind's existence, food scarcity was an existential issue. Unfortunately, this mentality is still part of our brain's heritage, imprinted in the most ancient part of our brain.[6]

Our brains are geared to prepare for a scarcity of energy-rich food sources. Today, for most people, access to inexpensive, ultra-processed foods are ever present. But our instincts, our DNA, still direct us, at some level, to eat whenever food is available, which is virtually always.

Cheap, high-calorie food is not only almost always available, the nature of the food we consume most often has fundamentally changed as well. As Dr. Andrew Weil points out in his book *Healthy Aging*, our foods changed from being unprocessed, unrefined, raw, natural and whole to highly processed, discarding the highest fiber parts of the food.[7] So our body metabolizes and breaks down these foods into glucose much more quickly, with unintended, associated negative consequences.

Innate Preference for High-Sugar Foods
Hominids and early Homo sapiens found that sweet foods were safe sources of energy that could be easily consumed without negative, unintended consequences and were quite rare in the natural environment.[8] Sugar also converts rapidly to the basic type of fuel used by our body and our cells, namely, glucose, to provide a quick jolt of energy. That is why we naturally love sweet, high-sugar foods, and our evolutionary history gives humans an innate predisposition and preference for sugary food sources and highly processed, simple carbs. Bitter, foul-tasting plants or berries

were more likely to make those who consumed them ill, or worse, might be poisonous.[9]

Before the era of hominids and early Homo sapiens, carbohydrates (except in fruits and vegetables) did not exist. Only in recent history have such highly processed foods evolved and rapidly proliferated (corresponding with the most rapid increase in the rate of obesity). Most of these highly processed, simple-carb foods contain a great deal of sugar. Because they taste so sweet we humans love and crave these highly processed foods.

Unfortunately, our bodies do not metabolize these highly processed foods in the same way as foods that are high in complex carbs and found in nature (like fruits and vegetables). These highly processed, foods break down into glucose (i.e., sugar) very quickly and cause our blood sugar levels to rise rapidly with associated negative consequences. When blood sugar spikes and later crashes back down, it typically results in our feeling hangry (see Chapter 22 for more about feeling hangry). And hangry feelings precipitate hunger and a craving for more high-sugar foods, resulting in overeating and weight gain. This whole premise is encapsulated in the in the theory behind the Glycemic Index.[10] Focusing on controlling and reducing your consumption of high-glycemic foods that either contain significant calories from sugar or are easily converted to sugar is an important key to weight loss and weight loss maintenance. The Whole Brain Diet Lifestyle offers a powerful and eminently useful way to counter and defuse the cravings you have for high-sugar, high-calorie foods, and the Take 5 technique is central to achieving this.

Factors Driving Obesity

Our instincts drive us to overeat, but, when food was very scarce and the energy, i.e., caloric expenditure, to obtain food was also extremely high, starvation was an operative challenge. Compare this to today's environment, now we say that we are "starving" not eating for all of seven to eight hours.

We must understand the two primal behavioral imperatives and realize that they may motivate us to engage in behaviors that in the world we face today are inconsistent with, and even counter to, the purpose of these ancient drives.[11] These instincts, which evolved and were reinforced over millions of years of evolutionary history, can lead us, via our subconscious, to overeat, binge and more generally eat an unhealthy diet.[12]

In just the past 60 years, the average daily intake of the American adult has increased by 570 calories (a 23 percent increase).[13] So, perhaps it is not shocking that the rate of obesity has tripled for men and doubled for women over the past 60 years. Interestingly, this is the same time period that corresponds with an explosion in the availability of highly processed simple carb foods and snacks.

Unconscious Impulses versus Conscious Deliberation

In his book *Thinking Fast and Slow,* Daniel Kahneman says that our deliberate, rational higher-level brain articulates judgments and makes decisions, but it often echoes or rationalizes ideas and feelings that were generated by the subconscious emotional parts of our brain. A very important inference is that our emotions and our instincts drive much of our behavior.[14] The Take 5 technique provides a shortcut to counter these instinctual emotional impulses that drive you to snack unhealthfully and to overeat. With effort, practice and perseverance, these impulses can be controlled.[15]

You need a strategy to bridge the period between initial intentions to create a new habit until it becomes firmly entrenched. This bridge strategy allows you to override your subconscious emotional *Fat* brain and prevent it from always ruling your behavior, while allowing the conscious intentions of your *Skinny* brain to be carried forward to fruition.

Creating a Whole Brain Diet Lifestyle

Rudy Tanzi and Deepak Chopra in their book *Super Brain*, contend that the primitive reactions of our brain are rarely appropriate in today's modern world. They persist as if humans still need to fight predators, fend off raiding tribes and run away from existential threats.[16] Humans also contended with the specter of food deprivation and real starvation. The brain's primal reactions are biologically hard-wired, but this does not mean that these drives must command your behavior. With the appropriate intentions, bolstered by enough willpower, you can utilize your self-control to override these instincts, and the Take 5 technique helps you to do exactly this.

What does this mean to designing a lifestyle for better, healthful eating in today's world? The Whole Brain Diet Lifestyle is firmly grounded on facing, understanding and then exploiting the real issues about the role and influence of the dual behavioral imperatives still operative in our brains today. An effective and healthy lifestyle plan includes constructing a total food environment to reduce your psychological, social and physical accessibility to poor quality foods. You must limit your opportunities for overeating or bingeing and minimize your unhealthful snacking. You should maximize the likelihood of reaching for and consuming a lower-calorie, nutrient-rich food. You cannot completely deny or eliminate your natural instincts to eat too much, too often or to enjoy high-sugar, high-calorie foods, but you can often counter them and redirect your impulses in a healthier and less fattening direction.

I give you the tools you need to utilize your brain to better manage your impulses and provide a long-term lifestyle you can employ for a healthier life. The Whole Brain Diet Lifestyle plan shows you how as Ben Franklin used to say, "to eat to live, not live to eat." While the plan offers many provocative ideas and highly specific behaviors and tools to facilitate a healthier lifestyle, it still projects an aura of common sense and authenticity that make it plausible and sustainable for a lifetime. The Take 5 technique is at the core of this plan by offering a simple tool everyone is capable of understanding and using. But the totality of the Whole Brain Diet Lifestyle comprises so much more.

I do not just recommend what changes in mind-set and behavior to implement, I tell you exactly how to make this plan actually work for you. This is a marked difference to many other self-help books, which tell you what to do, but not so much how to actually do it.

Another advantage is that you do not have to implement every suggestion. You can integrate into your life only those aspects that seem most sensible and viable for you to follow and adhere to. I offer alternative ways to arrive at the same goal of facilitating significant, transformational behavioral change in your life. Of course, the more of the total plan that you adopt the better, the better your chance of realizing a large and permanent change to your life.

If you implement the Whole Brain Diet Lifestyle plan, it naturally leads to healthier eating, a better, lower and more sustainable weight level, improved well-being and hence, a happier and (likely) longer life.

Let's now begin your journey toward a better and healthier diet lifestyle and ultimately a weightless state of being.

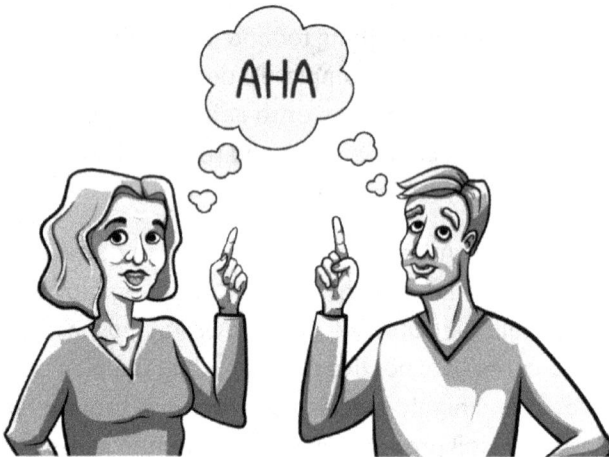

- Restricting your psychological, social and physical access to high-sugar and high-calorie foods is critical to weight control and to making real, long-run, dietary lifestyle changes. That is why constructing barriers to block their ready accessibility is so vital and why this is a major theme of this book.
- Our brains evolved for one primary purpose: to keep us alive long enough to procreate and care for our young. To our DNA, everything else, what we consider our life, is extraneous fluff. It's not that your life does not matter, just that to your DNA it is incidental to its real purpose, i.e., the perpetuation of our species. This is why it is so difficult to ignore the powerful signals emitted by your *Fat* brain as these signals in the early days of mankind were life and species preserving.

Part 1:

The Take 5 Technique

Chapter 1: Cravings and the Take 5 Technique

You can't eliminate your cravings, but you have the ability to not yield to them.

This chapter describes in detail the Take 5 technique. It is a very simple but powerful technique you can use to rapidly disarm your cravings. It is a method that readily and effectively disrupts an emotional impulse that might drive you to consume a high-sugar, high-calorie food at an unplanned or inappropriate time.

Your cravings originate in your brain. You cannot consciously, will your cravings to stop. They're instinctually and culturally driven. But if you have a means to rapidly shift your thinking and reactivity from a highly automatic and unconscious basis, to a slower, more deliberate conscious level, your cravings can be controlled. This way you can override and defuse your impulse to eat unhealthful snacks.

This was the genesis for developing Take 5. It acts as an emotional circuit breaker, which can be used to automatically initiate a pause before you respond to an emotional impulse. It's a method that allows you to handle a craving, the same craving that drives you to eat a high-sugar, high-calorie snack.

The Nature and Origin of Cravings

Your cravings serve a purpose. Cravings remind us to seek and consume food. Early Homo sapiens were not nuanced thinkers. Their pre-frontal cortex was highly underdeveloped. They didn't plan ahead, they acted on instinct and in the context of their immediate environment. In the early days of mankind, the connection between food, energy and survival was not understood. Cravings for food incentivized hominids to expend the energy and effort necessary to ensure that they ate enough to survive.

When we eat, the act of eating is reinforced by the release of the pleasurable neurochemical dopamine. Dopamine makes us feel good, making our brain happy, and our brains like to feel happy. No food delivers a more potent or rapid release of dopamine than sugar, as sugar (or technically glucose) is the basic energy source that powers the brain[1]. The brain can't store glucose or build up a reserve, so it needs to receive it regularly. Our cravings helped to incentivize early humans to seek and eat the food.

Very early in life, even as infants, we come to naturally associate food, especially high-sugar foods, with rewarding feelings. This preference for, and the drive to seek, high-sugar foods is facilitated by our cravings. However, in the days of early Homo sapiens food was scarce, as was the availability of sugar in the natural environment. Over-consumption of any food was a very rare event.

Cravings are powerful, but intriguing research from Dana Small of Yale University, offers a highly plausible explanation for why some cravings are so much more difficult to resist than others. His research suggests that when people are exposed to foods high in both carbs and fats, our ability to evaluate their nutritional value is impaired. Our ability to assess a food's nutritional value has a highly adaptive purpose, i.e., to help us to identify, seek and find high energy foods. But this innate ability goes awry with processed foods that are high in both carbs and fats. Small found that highly processed foods and snacks stimulate the brain's reward center significantly more than foods high in only carbs or fats. Further, the calorie content of such foods was consistently under-estimated and simultaneously, their nutritional value tended to be over-estimated.

Foods high in both carbs and fats were not readily available until the last 150 years with the advent of the first processed foods like potato chips and donuts. Our brains have not had enough time to adapt to the prevalence and high availability of processed foods. Today processed foods make-up about three-fifths of what Americans buy at the grocery store. It is hard to miss the correlation of the explosion of highly processed food availability over the past 60 years and the corresponding rapid rise in the rate of obesity.

It is also true that people who are overweight, especially if obese, are more likely to feel even greater anticipatory pleasure from eating high-carb, high-fat snack foods than other people. For these people, resisting a craving to eat this type of food is even more difficult than for those who are not overweight. Fortunately, the Take 5 technique mitigates these high-intensity cravings and is even more useful to weight-challenged people who need it the most.

In her seminal book, *How Emotions Are Made*, Lisa Feldman Barrett says, "Your brain's most important job is not thinking or feeling or even seeing, but keeping your body alive and well so that you survive and thrive." This is why your unconscious self, the part that allows you to react automatically when you face a threat is so powerful. Your unconscious self always remains vigilant and ready to act very rapidly with little or any conscious thought. This is why the emotionally impulsive cravings that originate in your unconscious mind are so forceful and so hard to resist and this is why Take 5 is so very useful.

Take 5 is exactly the assist our brains need to counter the extraordinary anticipatory pleasure and resulting burst of feel-good dopamine generated by the thought of eating these high-carb, high-fat foods. Cravings are very hard to resist and Take 5 was designed to rapidly defuse them. This is the core of the Whole Brain Diet Lifestyle plan.

You can help yourself by striving to configure your environment to reduce and to avoid the cues that trigger your cravings, which release an emotional impulse to eat unhealthy snacks. For example, you should:

- Keep all high-sugar and highly processed simple-carb foods out of sight to reduce their physical and psychological accessibility.
- Keep low-calorie, low-sugar and nutrient-dense snacks always visible and readily accessible.
- Minimize viewing the cable TV cooking shows, with their incredibly tempting and indulgent desserts.
- Avoid reading magazines that are filled with tempting food images and easy-to-follow dessert recipes.
- Always eat a substantial, whole-food breakfast. It should contain either high-complex-carbs, high-fiber, and or high-protein that fills the belly for a long time.
- Always keep visual mantras like the statement "eat smart – eat in moderation" in your line of sight.

The Take 5 Technique

These steps help to reduce exposure to the precipitating factors that trigger your cravings but not eliminate them, and this is where Take 5 becomes extremely useful. A central focus is to make you more self-aware and more mindful by following the Whole Brain Diet Lifestyle. The Take 5 technique is a very powerful and a very easy method you can use to operationalize the concept of mindfulness. This allows you to naturally counter and mitigate the cravings that drive you to overeat. After you first experience a new craving, you can activate the Take 5 technique by taking the following 8-steps:

Step 1: Tell yourself to Take 5, e.g., say "(*Your Name*), Take 5."

Step 2: Commit to wait five minutes before you respond to the craving and simultaneously move yourself to a different location from where you experienced the craving.

Step 3: Exhale deeply, then slowly take a very deep breath in for four seconds (through your nose), hold it for four seconds, and then breathe out for eight seconds (through your mouth and purse your lips for maximum exhalation) while silently repeating a mantra like, "Patience Now," "I Got This," or perhaps "Serenity Now" (thank you to Frank Costanza on Seinfeld for those iconic words). Then repeat this exercise four more times. While inhaling, simultaneously breathe in a scent from a vial of a calming oil like lavender, lemon or chamomile (a useful, but optional step.)

Step 4: Drink an ice-cold glass of water.

Step 5: Label the feeling you experienced as a craving and think about:

How does it make your body and your mind feel, i.e., how would you describe it to someone else?

How intense was the feeling?

Is the feeling true physical hunger or simply an emotional response?

What might have been the cue(s) that precipitated the craving and how can you minimize being exposed to these cues in the future?

Step 6: Repeat to yourself (or out loud). "(*Your Name*) is feeling a craving to eat an unhealthy, high-sugar snack, but, he/she has the power to make a choice to yield or not to yield to this craving, and he/she chooses not to."

Step 7: Vividly use your imagination to conjure up an image of you eating the snack you were craving while relaxing on the beach on a beautiful, sunny day, or imagine any place that you find very relaxing.

Step 8: Use any remaining time to calm, soothe and quiet your mind.

In Step 1, you are simply announcing to yourself your intention to Take 5. This is where you start to initiate a shift in perspective, that is, a shift in your mind-set, from your normal, virtually automatic and unconscious response, to a more deliberate and conscious response mode.

Step 2 helps to create both a psychological and physical distance from where the craving arose, and, if you were in the kitchen (where many cravings do originate), it also helps to provide a physical distance from the specific snack temptation. In some ways, using Take 5 is like imposing a time out on a child. The first rule is to remove the child (or in this case, yourself) from a reinforcing environment (like the kitchen or TV room) to a less reinforcing environment to decrease the undesirable behavior. When you do this, you blunt the impact of the emotional impulse to eat an unhealthful snack.

In Step 3, the first specific action called for is to breathe deeply in and out. Inhale, hold and exhale, this pattern activates your parasympathetic nervous system, and automatically slows down your heart rate and helps to relax your body and mind.[2] Further, inhaling the aromatic essential oils goes right to your brain directly, without intermediation from any other sensory organ. This creates an immediate state of relaxation and less stress, making it far easier to be patient and wait a full five minutes to give your craving time to dissipate.

In Step 4, drinking a glass of water has multiple benefits. It reduces the momentum moving you to yield to your craving. Also, your craving may actually be driven by thirst as much or more than your actually being hungry. Finally, drinking a glass of water also helps to fill the belly, making eating something, anything, a little less appealing.

Step 5 helps you in a couple of ways. First, it helps you to understand and learn what factors trigger the cues that activate your cravings. Understanding these precipitating factors helps you to avoid or minimize them in the future, as well as to reduce their future intensity. Second, the simple act of describing and labeling a feeling reduces the emotional urgency of the moment, making it easier to wait the whole five minutes before acting. Third, it gives you something constructive to do during your five-minute pause that also distracts you from the initial craving impulse.

Also, in Step 5, the act of labeling and describing a feeling or emotion reduces its intensity, which lessens the momentum propelling you to behave without thinking. In many cases, you will find that when you actually stop to analyze what you are feeling, it is not real hunger. It often is a negative emotional state, such as anger, frustration, tension or even boredom that precipitated the craving to eat. These emotions are best addressed not by eating, but by accepting, resolving the emotion and letting it go. It is the passage of time, plus the act of introspection, that shifts your thinking into a conscious, deliberate mode where you can make an informed decision to eat or not eat a snack.

In Step 6, a reinforcing statement crystallizes your intention to not yield to the craving. It may feel a little odd to frame the statement in the third person, but research supports its value. University of Michigan scientists explain that the neuropsychological effect of talking to yourself in the third person helps to control your emotions. Talking to yourself in the third person is a simple and cognitively inexpensive (i.e., not mentally taxing) way to reduce negative emotions on the spot.[3]

In Step 7, you use your imagination to envision consuming a high-sugar snack. Research indicates that this act results in the anticipatory release of the feel-good neurotransmitter dopamine. No, it's not exactly the same jolt of dopamine as eating the sugary snack releases, but it is real and produces a positive feeling. As Robert Sapolsky says in his book *Behave,* "often we are more about the anticipation and pursuit of pleasure than about the experience of it."[4] Although it may be counterintuitive, it is often true, and you can use this reality to your advantage in helping to make the Take 5 method work for you.

In Step 8, by utilizing any remaining time to calm and quiet your mind, your stress is reduced even more, helping to further mitigate the craving impulse that you are experiencing and lower your likelihood of consuming an unhealthful snack.

After five minutes elapse, in many instances the craving dissipates and is unlikely to return any time soon. If the urge or craving to eat is still present, you are in a position to engage and use your deliberate conscious thinking mode to decide how to react. You can decide to:

- Seek and consume a healthier low-sugar, low-calorie, nutrient-dense snack like a piece of fruit, vegetable or (low-sugar) yogurt.
- Eat a very small portion of high-sugar, high-calorie snack that you wisely pre-portioned for just this possibility.
- Resolve to wait for one additional five-minute period to see if the craving finally goes away for good.

If you do decide to have a high-sugar snack, you can eat a very small pre-portioned size. Your snack craving can often be satisfied even by indulging in just a few small bites.[5] Your brain releases the biggest jolt of dopamine after just the first few bites of a sugary snack, and it diminishes after that.[6] You will be surprised how often a very small sweet snack satisfies you.

In any case, the decision is consciously and deliberatively chosen, instead of a semi-automatic, reflexive response. Using the Take 5 technique reduces the snacks, which you did not deliberately decide to consume. Serendipitously, you also enjoy the good feeling that comes with, as Rudy Tanzi likes to say, being the "user of your brain, not its unwitting subject."

Take 5 is an excellent and highly useful tool in the era of the Coronavirus. Any time you are home your access to junk food is increased, but during the enhanced home confinement due to the Coronavirus your access is at an extreme level. Take 5 can help. My family and extended family have all employed it to help reduce the likelihood that they reach for and eat, or overeat, unhealthy, high-sugar, high-calorie junk foods. Here's one story to illustrate this point. My granddaughters, stressed by their self-confinement and bored from too little stimulation, were about to reach for another junk food snack. Their mother, my daughter, said to the girls, "Girl's Take 5." And she asked them to take a 5-minute pause and reassess whether or not they were truly hungry, or merely, stressed and bored. The girls, familiar with the Take 5 method, paused, and, after a few minutes they went off without eating another snack. Take 5 can work as simply and quickly as that.

Here is another perfect example of using Take 5 from my own life. Not long ago, my wife and I went out to for a expensive dinner. While still eating, I saw a waiter wheel the dessert cart over to another table. It was filled with wonderful and mouth-watering concoctions. I was quite full and feeling satisfied, but the thought of one of those desserts was setting my brain's reward center on fire. I knew I was vulnerable and decided to employ a Take 5 pause. I said to myself, *Ken, Take 5.* I paused, reflected and asked myself, *is the fleeting pleasure of eating a dessert, worth the hundreds of additional calories and the uncomfortable feeling of an overstuffed belly.* We all know the feeling, despite being full, when you still indulge anyway in a restaurant-sized, super-rich and heavy dessert. Immediately afterward, you feel uncomfortable, even queasy and nauseous, and you ask yourself, "Why did I do that, it was so unnecessary." I did not suffer this regret, as after our meal, when the waiter approached with the dessert cart, after employing a Take 5 pause, I easily said, "No, thank you."

"Punctuated Eating" and Take 5

One very innovative way to use Take 5 is to make it an integral part of a leisurely, mealtime eating process. I call this process "punctuated eating." It involves using alternating periods of 5-minute Take 5 pauses and 5-minutes of eating in a manner that makes overeating much less likely. The process works as follows:

- Employ a 5-minute Take 5 pause to focus your mind on eating slowly, mindfully and savoring every bite.
- Use the next 5-minutes to start eating, being sure to eat slowly and mindfully and taking a mini-pause in eating by putting your utensil down between every bite.
- Take a second 5-minute, Take 5 pause to imagine yourself enjoying your food and stopping eating when you feel merely satisfied, not completely full.
- Eat for an additional 5-minute period, again, taking your time to enjoy and savor every bite.
- Take a third and final 5-minute Take 5 pause to sense the increasing fullness in your belly, sense yourself becoming more satisfied and sense yourself approaching satiety.
- End your meal with 5-minutes of slow, mindful eating.

There are several benefits to this "punctuated eating" process:

- You learn how to naturally and easily sense yourself slowly getting fuller and more satisfied.

- You learn to stop eating when you feel satisfied and before you feel totally full or stuffed. As a result, you eat less, consume fewer calories and are less likely to overeat.
- Spending 30-minutes over your meal physically gives your body time to reach a real state of satiation and this can keep help to keep your mind alert and focused for hours on matters of your choosing.
- You are likely to actually enjoy eating your food more without the post-meal discomfort you feel if you overeat.

Innovative Take 5 Application

Another innovative application for employing Take 5 can greatly strengthen your capacity to disarm your snack cravings and has unexpected power to aid you in your goal to reduce high-calorie snacking. Twice a day, engage in a Take 5 exercise where you imagine that you are experiencing a craving to eat your favorite unhealthful snack and not yielding to the temptation. That's it! The imaginary act strengthens the neurons in your brain associated with this act making it more likely that when you do feel a real-world high-sugar craving you are able to resist it. Neuroscientists like to say, "The neurons that fire together, wire together." This creates your default response when these same neurons are activated by a similar stimuli.

When you are faced with the choice to eat or not to eat a high-sugar, high-calorie snack it creates a state of cognitive dissonance in your mind that needs to be resolved. Your emotional unconscious wants to enjoy the sweet taste, while your conscious self knows it's not healthful. The more often you choose to not yield to a sweet snack temptation, the more this action becomes automatic. It allows you to bypass relying on your willpower and to drive your response by habit.

The more you practice the Take 5 technique, the more natural and automatic it becomes. Repeat the following statement every day until the technique is automatically activated when you experience a craving and the Take 5 method becomes habitual. Say to yourself:

"(*Your Name*) Takes 5 any time he/she feels a craving to snack on a high-sugar, high-calorie food. It's a great way to ensure that (*Your Name*) 'eats smart – eats in moderation.' (*Your Name*) knows that his/her brain is the master of his/her behavior and that he/she is the master of his/her brain."

You should also strive to turn the phrase "Take 5" into a self-induced mantra that becomes lodged in your consciousness. In addition to repeating this statement, you can help to create this meme by obtaining and wearing a wristband that simply says in bold letters: **TAKE 5**. The goal is to help make your usage of the Take 5 method so routine that it becomes a habit, something you automatically do when you experience a craving to eat high-sugar, high-calorie foods.

You should also tell your spouse/partner/friends about Take 5. They can not only benefit from it as well, but their awareness helps support your own intention and resolve to use it. If they also choose to use the Take 5 technique, it provides a great natural reinforcement for your own continued usage.

Another innovative way to make using Take 5 natural and habitual for me, was what I call, "Take 5 to Take 5." Once a day, I actually used the Take 5 technique to engage in slow, rhythmic in and out breathing while silently repeating the words Take 5. While inhaling through my nose I said to myself the word "Take" and during my exhale through my mouth I said to myself the word "5." This process helped me to imprint onto my brain the idea of using Take 5. Today, Take 5 is an integral part of my life and I no longer need to engage it for this specific purpose.

At the end of every day, perhaps right before bedtime, you should review how well you achieved your goal to eat smart – eat in moderation and how well using Take 5 helped you to do this. If you did not do very well that day, think about why and what you might have done differently. Tell yourself, "Tomorrow is a new day and a new chance to use Take 5 to pursue my goal to eat smart – eat in moderation."

Another factor driving the successful utilization of Take 5 is your instinct for survival. Your instincts evolved so that your natural state of being is to spend the least amount of energy for the most amount of reward.[7] The energy needed to implement Take 5 is very low, and the reward for its usage is very high. This makes Take 5 easy to adopt and easy to follow.

University of Pennsylvania psychologist Angela Duckworth said, "When a goal is important to you and costs to achieve it are low and the likelihood of success is high, it leads to goal accomplishment."[8] The goal of eating smart and in moderation is highly important. The "cost" of using the Take 5 method requires only a small expenditure of mental and physical energy. This makes it easier to incorporate Take 5 into your daily routine.

The ultimate goal of practicing the Take 5 technique and the highest level of Whole Brain Diet Lifestyle attainment that you can reach, is when you no longer even need to consciously invoke it and use it for snack deterrence. When you automatically and habitually eat smart – eat in moderation, your cravings permanently diminish, and you no longer are a slave to your emotional impulses, you are weightless.

As a final thought, it is worth noting that the Take 5 method has much broader applicability than for just handling food cravings. It can be used in virtually any situation where you can benefit by employing an emotional circuit breaker to defuse negative emotional stimuli and allow it to lessen or even dissipate completely. The next chapter explores some of the other applications for which Take 5 may be highly useful.

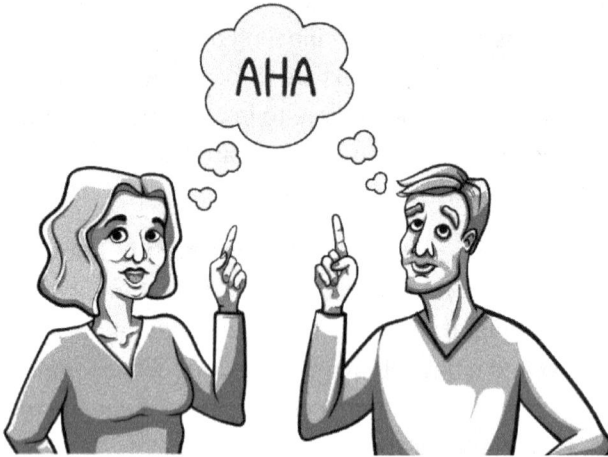

- The logic supporting the merits and value of the Take 5 technique has scientific and common-sense validity as an emotional circuit breaker.
- When you use the Take 5 technique enough for it to become routine and habitual, you automatically help to defuse the natural innate tension between your *Fat* brain and your *Skinny* brain in a manner that is sustainable for a lifetime.

Chapter 2: More Take 5 Applications
When You Make Take 5 a Part of Your Daily Life, it Changes Your Life in Unexpected Ways.

I developed the Take 5 technique with the specific intent to create a tool suited to deter and thwart the cravings to snack and to overeat. But I soon realized that Take 5 was a tool that could be used to combat and defuse virtually any negative impulse or negative emotional state and allow it to dissipate much more quickly than without any intervention. I realized that any time you wanted or needed to calm down, reduce your stress and/or reboot and re-energize your brain, Take 5 was an applicable tool.

Regularly using Take 5 can have a positive spill over into other aspects of your lifestyle, a halo effect. When you are able to thwart your cravings it serendipitously increases your feelings of mastery and efficacy. These feelings give you the confidence and incentive to tackle other parts of your lifestyle that you desire to change and improve.

One way to classify the many additional, potential applications of Take 5 is to view it in terms of the specific scenario in which it is being employed. It can be used in situations involving just you, or with yourself and other people such as your spouse/partner/lover, parents, children, colleagues and your friends. In any circumstance where you are in need of a regulator to mitigate an emotionally charged situation or defuse a negative impulse, Take 5 can be invoked and usefully employed.

Why and how does Take 5 work? Well, one neuroscientist provided a clue when she said that everyone has a choice, "moment to moment to choose what we do and who we are."[1] This is the absolute essence of mindfulness and the deep, core basis for how and why Take 5 works. Take 5 is an excellent tool to bring you rapidly into a state of mindful awareness allowing you to make a discrete choice on how you respond.

Another important reason that you are likely to integrate Take 5 into your life is that the human brain is lazy. It always strives to conserve mental and physical energy, so shortcuts are often favored to solve a problem. Take 5 provides exactly this type of shortcut as you can very rapidly invoke it and use it to address many different scenarios. As Take 5 becomes more habitual, it evolves into being your go-to shortcut to address any situation where your goal is to mitigate and defuse a negative emotional impulse.

Situations for Which Take 5 is Well-Suited

Take 5 is well-suited to situations where you are experiencing a wide variety of emotions including any of the following:

- Anger or rage
- Fear
- Frustration
- Boredom
- Nervousness
- Impatience
- Procrastination
- Melancholy
- Hyperactivity
- Anxiety

When you feel any of these emotions, call upon Take 5 to help break their momentum. When you pause, think and introspect, you may realize that there is often no recognizable basis for legitimately feeling this way, it is simply a passing state of mind generated by internal bodily sensations. By breathing deeply, pausing and introspecting, you can calm the body, let go of a negative emotion and allow it to dissipate and float away.

Many stimuli invoke a feeling of fear and a great urge to respond to that fear immediately. This is especially true when one is as technologically challenged as myself. One day when I was writing this book, I experienced, metaphorically speaking, an existential fear provoking event. Suddenly, without warning my screen froze and there appeared in dramatic large red letters a threat, "Your computer is at immediate risk of being infected with a malicious virus that will destroy and delete ALL the files on your hard drive. Click here NOW to prevent this." My computer had my only copy of my manuscript and I was momentarily frozen in fear. What should I do? My response was to Take 5. I paused and thought to myself, "Ken, this is probably a scam for money." Or worse, I reasoned if I actually clicked on the button, that itself might cause a virus to enter my computer and take it over. This actually happened to a close family friend, and his panicky, unconscious fear ended up costing him nearly $1,000 to rectify.

By engaging my conscious, deliberate response mode, I was able to break the momentum driving me to toward an immediate and possibly irreversible action. I reasoned that if I simply shutdown and subsequently rebooted the computer, I could safely see what would happen. Worse case the red alert would reappear, perhaps signifying that it was in fact a legitimate warning. So, I shutdown, the alert did not reappear. Take 5 worked exactly as I hoped. The 5-minute pause allowed me to engage my conscious, deliberate, reasoning self and think through the potential consequences of taking one action or another.

Here is another example where Take 5 can be helpful when you encounter a situation that raises a fear of an actual physical threat, even if that threat is totally imaginary. One winter's night I was walking in my neighborhood on a dark and empty street. Approaching me in the shadows were two men I didn't recognize. While they towered above in statute, they were not menacing, yelling or gesturing to me at all; yet I was fearful. I tried to recall what I had learned about our evolutionary instincts. I knew that we humans are innately predisposed to be suspicious and fearful of those who appear to be different from us or who are not part of our clan. This alert in the early days of Homo sapiens armed you to flee or fight those who might wish to harm you, but, in this age, merely serve to unnecessarily frighten you. I needed a means to engage my conscious, reasoning self and I found just that by employing Take 5. I told myself, "Ken, your fear is unjustified and not grounded in any reality; calm down and keep on walking." I did just that and as they came closer to me they greeted me with a smile and a hello. Take 5 helped me to disengage from and counter my natural evolutionarily-based fears and behave in a manner consistent with my intentions.

Since I developed the Take 5 technique, I have had many occasions to use it to help myself and others. One fundamentally valuable application that is highly useful in any of these venues is to employ Take 5 to disrupt an impulse to say or do something unkind. If you feel an impulse to be unkind, you should tell yourself, "(*Your Name*), Take 5." Then breathe deeply, consciously pause and ask yourself, does this unkind act really further your goals, will it be useful to you in some real way, or is it unnecessary and likely to merely be destructive? Most likely, the impulse to be unkind simply passes without your feeling the need to act on it.

In-Home Applications for Take 5

At home, Take 5 can be used to defuse negative and potentially unpleasant interactions with your spouse, partner, children or parents. When one of these people pushes your buttons and says or does something inflammatory that could easily escalate into an argument, even a shouting match, Take 5. Breathe deeply, pause and make a conscious choice to have a real dialogue, not a fight.

One of the most useful reasons to Take 5 is to mitigate angry feelings. My wife is a very passionate person with strong opinions. But since employing Take 5, our heated exchanges have mellowed and subsided a bit. My wife uses Take 5 to limit how often she expresses her own outspoken passions. I use it as well, so now when my wife does get angry, my own response is subdued. The result is that we cut off a potentially extended angry exchange before it can escalate unpleasantly. For us, using Take 5 is a win-win scenario.

With your children, when they say or do something you find inappropriate or objectionable, you can simply tell them and yourself to Take 5. This gives some time for all of you to chill out. The contentious moment likely passes, and you may be able to move on without saying or doing something regretful.

Everyone wants to avoid unnecessary family acrimony with your spouse or children or even your grandchildren. Here is an example of how I used Take 5 in a situation with my granddaughters. Living very close to my two granddaughters is one of the greatest joys of my life. I love them very dearly and unconditionally. But they are three years apart and can bicker and argue incessantly and unmercifully.

One evening, when their parents were out, I was watching over them. Euphemistically, I told myself that I was in charge, although in reality this was illusionary. On this occasion, their hostility and shouting reached an unbearable crescendo and I felt myself losing it. I feared I would say or do something inappropriate to restore peace. Thankfully, instead, I merely told myself, "Ken, Take 5." I paused, breathed deeply and reminded myself that these girls were simply young and immature, not bad people who needed to be punished. I contemplated what a better and more successful approach might be.

My reasoned response, in a soft and calm manner was to tell them, "Girls, Pop-Pop is very unhappy with your loud bickering, it is giving me a headache." I said to them, "I would be very appreciative if you would both calm down. If you cannot play together in peace, go to your rooms and play by yourself." Then I said, "Girls, you need to Take 5, take 5-minutes to think about your behavior and how you want to proceed." That was all that I needed to do. Lashing out in anger would only have exacerbated the tensions and unhappiness. By employing Take 5, I was able to shift my response mode from an unconscious angry state to a conscious state where I could calm down and follow a commonsense course of action. To defuse intense emotions in both yourself and others, Take 5 is a great tool.

In-Office Applications for Take 5

At the office, a colleague might say something you find offensive or hurtful, and you feel like responding in kind. A better choice is to Take 5 and let the negative impulse dissipate. Or maybe a colleague wants to engage in some petty and inappropriate gossiping. Just Take 5 and resist the urge to become complicit. Many colleagues may subject you to a barrage of negativity about your workplace or your boss. Simply Take 5 before you respond. Your instinct to be sociable might drive you to engage in this type of negativity, but it's seldom a productive use of your time.

Perhaps you are by yourself and you are stuck in a rut without any new ideas to solve a problem. If you Take 5, you can calmly reboot and re-energize your brain, uncluttering it to attack the problem with renewed vigor. Using Take 5 helps you to cut through the brain fog we all are occasionally subject to and refresh your mind. In fact, any time you need to concentrate intently, you can Take 5 to clear your mind and boost your ability to focus.

Also, you might get a bit nervous about leading a meeting or presenting to a group at work. In these situations, Take 5 is a great tool to help you calm down, destress, focus and collect your thoughts. It can also help you to reframe and actually transform this nervousness into a catalyst you can harness productively to energize your meeting or your presentation.

Any time you are challenged with a difficult issue with multiple conflicting solutions, you can Take 5. Give yourself some time to really consider all of the alternatives and not just the first ones that come to your mind or are consistent with your pre-existing beliefs. Take 5 allows you to pause and think about the fact that your first solution is often not the optimal one. Take 5 provides a means to help cut through the confirmation bias that causes you to seek and accept beliefs and solutions that are familiar to you and to consider more original solutions that might perform much better.

You can also employ the Take 5 technique in a social venue when you feel an impulse to respond without enough deliberate conscious thought. Everyone has said something in a social setting that they immediately regretted the moment they said it. Take 5 mitigates some inappropriate or potentially embarrassing behavior that taking some deep breaths and a pause helps you avoid.

Some time ago, my wife and I went out to breakfast with very old friends whose different political leanings were straining our friendship. We knew if the conversation devolved into politics, sparks could fly, tempers would flare, and hurtful words might be exchanged. We greatly valued the friendship and resolved to steer clear of any temptation to engage them in political talk, as we all had entrenched beliefs and opinions that were not likely to be changed.

This particular morning when our friends strayed into talking about presidential politics, my wife and I knew where this might be heading, we looked each other in the eyes and silently repeated to ourselves, "Take 5." No, we did not pause speechless for a full five minutes. We defused our instinct to react, attack and promote our own brand of politics and we immediately steered the conversation to a neutral, safe topic.

Wherever you might be, in any circumstance where you find yourself, listening to and attending to the negative chatter in your mind, e.g., "What can go wrong?" "Why am I so inept?" or "How will I get through this?" you should Take 5. By breathing deeply, pausing and introspecting, you can break the cycle of negative chatter. As Rudy Tanzi and Deepak Chopra postulated in their book *Super Brain*, your thoughts are merely fleeting mental constructs without import unless, or until, you choose to attend to them. With Take 5 you can learn to listen to this chatter without judgment and let the negativity simply pass without attending to it.

Take 5 - Not Just an Intervention for Negative Emotions
You can train your brain to respond with a primarily negative or positive orientation, you have the choice. Why not choose positivity? It feels better and is more satisfying in the long-run. The regular, systematic use of Take 5 counters your negative impulses and allows your positivity to emerge. Over

time as your use of Take 5 becomes more automatic, your emotional default mode becomes more positive and less negative. The more you respond in a positive fashion, the more likely your brain is to do so again in similar circumstances.

Another very positive use of Take 5 as a cue is to engage in a nightly routine before going to bed. I recommend that you use the Take 5 pause to reflect and perhaps record in a journal:

- Compassionate thoughts directed toward yourself and others.
- At least five things you are grateful for that day.
- How you can best serve the needs of others in the days to come.

Research suggests that these activities make your life more purposeful and happier, resulting in a higher state of well-being.

Take 5 has real value beyond its role in disrupting and defusing negative emotional impulses and improve your physical health. As you use Take 5 over time, it gives you an increasing sense of control over your life. This heightened sense of control naturally leads to reduced feelings of stress, which has a positive impact on your health. Reduced stress increases your feelings of eudaimonia well-being, which causes a downward regulation of the genes that trigger inflammation in your body.[2] Inflammation is a fundamental cause of many chronic medical conditions, including heart disease and even dementia like Alzheimer's.

How to Make Take 5 More Effective

You can take some specific actions to amplify and optimize the effects of Take 5. For example, you can employ the power of positive expectations by repeating to yourself statements like:

> "Take 5 is a very powerful tool to disrupt negative emotional impulses. Take 5 always works for (*Your Name*)."
> "When (*Your Name*) needs a pause, a mental break, Take 5 works for him/her."

You can use Take 5 not only on an as needed basis, but also on a prescheduled basis, say every few hours. The systematic practice of Take 5 makes its usage more natural, more automatic and subsequently make it work even more quickly. Take 5 puts your conscious self in charge, improving your life and well-being.

The Bottom Line

Take 5 can be so much more than a specific technique to counter your snack cravings and to help regulate your emotions. It can be a philosophy for how to live your life harmoniously in a steadier emotional equilibrium, by curbing the unconsciously generated emotional impulses that stealthily and unwittingly impact your behavior in so many negative ways. As the eminent doctor and new-age philosopher Deepak Chopra said, "When you feel reactive, observe your reaction, in the pause between your conditioned responses there is spontaneous creativity."

The Take 5 technique is immensely powerful, incredibly versatile and highly effective. If you choose to use it for all, or many, of the circumstances where it is appropriate, it materially changes your life and improves your health and well-being. **Make Take 5 part of your daily life and it will transform your life for the better!**

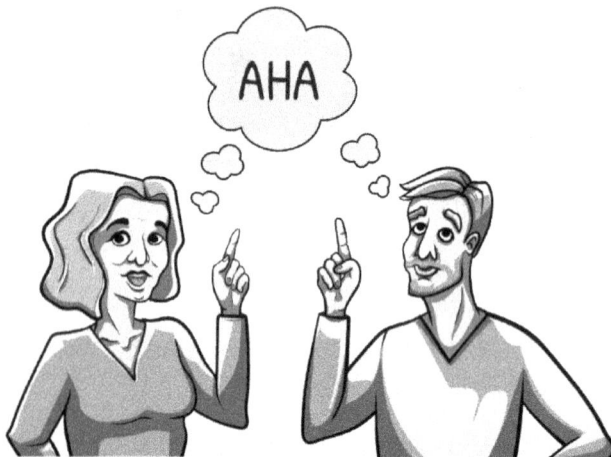

- Simply by using Take 5 regularly, you can train your brain in a fashion that makes using Take 5 more automatic and efficacious.
- When you use Take 5 with friends, family and colleagues and they start to adopt it as well, you reap its benefits by merely invoking the Take 5 mantra even before you complete the process. When you announce that you are going to Take 5, it becomes a communication shortcut that over time instantaneously demonstrates your intentions.

Part 2:

The Whole Brain Diet Lifestyle

Chapter 3: Why Is Weight Loss So Difficult?

You can't follow the same course of action with every diet and expect a different long-term outcome. Real lifestyle change is required.

Why Does Weight Accumulate Over Time?

Recent data established that as defined by the BMI (Body Mass Index), approximately 40 percent of the adult population is obese and over 70 percent are considered overweight.[1] Survey data also indicates that around 50 percent of adults are considering losing weight and a significant percentage of adults (25 percent) are actively on a diet.[2] Many people are overweight not due to a lack of awareness of their condition or a lack of intention to lose weight. It is related to how difficult long-run weight loss really is to accomplish.

If people know that being obese makes you both less attractive and less healthy and that obesity is a very tough challenge to overcome, why do they let the weight accumulate without taking action? It goes back to the fact that having a layer of fat is evolutionarily-favored as life preserving. The brain wants to be prepared for when food energy sources are very scarce, and fat provides a margin of safety that could be the difference between life and death. Keep in mind that for the vast majority of time since the emergence of Homo sapiens, humans were hunter-gatherers with an uncertain and scarce food supply. An abundance of food is an extremely recent occurrence.

It seems likely that humans are primed, unconsciously, to find some weight gain to be reassuring, even comforting. We may know intellectually that the weight is unnecessary and unattractive, but subconsciously we favor it. By the time our conscious brain signals we have gained too much weight, we may already be obese, and the self-perpetuating cycle is then very difficult to break.

Losing Weight

Almost everyone knows that weight loss is achieved primarily in only two ways. Either you decrease the number of calories digested and/or or materially increase the number of calories expended. There are also other issues as to why losing weight over the long-run is so hard.

Almost every diet leads to weight loss if followed, as virtually all diets encompass consuming fewer calories. Eat fewer calories than you expend, and you will lose weight. Some diets fail because they are boring and/or so restrictive that following them is too difficult to continue for long enough to achieve an acceptable weight loss. Some diets are so alien to our natural routines as to be unsustainable. Other weight-loss diets are easier to adhere to and work for some people for a while, but almost all of these fail over the long-run (i.e., over a 12-24 month period after the initial weight loss).[3] Why is this true?

Weight-loss diets are by their nature temporary. They change eating behavior only while they are actively followed. After the diet ends, most people go back to their pre-diet behavior. Of course, they (slowly perhaps) regain the weight lost. But there are other fundamental reasons why we regain the weight we lose.

Natural Mind-Body Reaction to Weight Loss

Research out of Mount Sinai hospital in New York provides even more evidence that traditional diet and exercise alone may not be enough to affect long-term weight loss.[4] The body naturally reacts to preserve your weight and even slows down a dieter's metabolism to expend fewer calories. This means that after you lose significant weight, you need fewer calories to maintain that weight than someone else who never underwent the same weight loss.[5]

Not only are most diets temporary, they actually activate forces that counter their effects. To lose weight and keep it off requires real modifications to your lifestyle including changes in what you eat, how you eat, how much you eat and how many calories you expend.

Our biology also conspires against our maintaining weight loss in another fundamental way. Research indicates that by our mid-20s we forever maintain all of the fat cells we have in our body. These fat cells may expand or shrink in size, but they do not ever go away. They are always available to absorb nutrients to make them larger and promote weight gain.[6] Unfortunately, eating not only makes your brain happy, it also makes your fat cells happy as well.

Another discouraging research finding indicates the direction of causality between eating, movement and obesity is bidirectional. Not only does eating more and moving less contribute to obesity; but once obese, the natural tendency is to eat more and move less.[7] A negative feedback loop is created that tends to help perpetuate obesity. Once established, this cycle is very difficult to break.

Why Timing and Preparation Matters

Diets also fail because inadequate attention is given to timing and preparation. All diet books and books devoted to dietary lifestyle change give you advice on what to do to achieve your weight or lifestyle change goals. Few if any, however, discuss timing parameters and why they matter. Most books tell you to follow their plan, their advice, but simply assume you will initiate your quest for change when you feel ready. But there is a much better, a more scientifically and common sense validated approach to the issue of when to begin. As Dan Pink says in his book, *When: The Scientific Secrets of Perfect Timing*, "Timing isn't everything, everything is timing."

There are a number of issues concerning the optimal timing for starting a program to lose weight and transform your dietary lifestyle. Nothing is more important than to consider the impact of evolutionary factors. A provocative British study showed that evolution programmed humans to store fat during the winter months when food is typically scarcer and less readily accessible.[8] Combining this with the fact that winter weather conditions and fewer daylight hours dissuade you from exercising outdoors, and it is apparent that starting a major weight reduction program or dietary lifestyle change on January 1 (as a New Year's Resolution) may possibly be the absolute worst time to begin. Nature is conspiring against successful weight loss and dietary change during the winter months, and I say, "Why fight Mother Nature?"

Research also suggests that the human brain works a little less efficiently, purposefully and effectively during the winter months and its performance peaks in the summer.[9] This is one more reason to delay initiating a major dietary behavioral change until spring has sprung. Human brains started to evolve in the always warm climate of the African continent and did not face truly cold weather until mankind began their migration out of Africa. Our brains love warm weather!

Bottom-line trying to initiate a major weight loss regimen during the winter is very difficult. Instead, a worthy goal is to simply try to maintain your weight and not gain while you wait for a more opportune time to start a major weight loss program. In addition to holding your weight steady and not digging yourself into a deeper hole, you start making Take 5 a part of your life.

It makes a lot of sense to link your initial efforts to following the Whole Brain Diet Lifestyle to a date of great traditional or personal significance. An excellent time to start following the plan is on the first weekend day after the beginning of the spring season. This is a time of the reawakening of nature and when we ourselves throw off the lethargy and sluggishness associated with winter. The lengthening of daylight hours and the warming of the sun energizes our spirit and intent. More importantly perhaps, this gives you nine months until the next winter season to establish the Whole Brain Diet Lifestyle as a routine you can follow habitually with little conscious effort.

Of course, it may be early winter when you feel highly motivated to initiate a fundamental change to your dietary lifestyle. It isn't sensible to simply shrug your shoulders and put it off until spring, which might be an additional ten pounds away. Instead start on your new diet lifestyle with the intent of just striving to maintain your weight. Use the winter months to begin to establish more healthful eating. Then, come the spring, you can hit the ground running, with your mind and body primed to initiate a major overhaul to your diet lifestyle.

It is easier to lose weight when we can be outdoors and our bodymind "knows" instinctually that food energy sources are more abundant. This feeling is still imprinted in our unconscious. Although it seems to no longer apply in the modern world where fruits and vegetables are abundantly available all year long, it is still operative. This feeling means that our bodymind is less inclined to unconsciously "hoard" calories by reducing our metabolism and our expenditure of energy. This, of course, makes losing weight harder in the winter months.

I suggest choosing a weekend (when most of us are not working) as the first day of your new dietary/lifestyle program. This gives you two days of typically less stressful time to get under way, two days when the demands on your mental and physical energy are lessened, making it easier to sustain your willpower and self-control. Even better is to begin during a staycation, a vacation you spend at home, away from the hurried lunches at work and the inevitable stress induced, snack-attack temptations.

Of course, in the era of the Coronavirus, if you are among those confined to home, you are in an extended staycation. One without the temptations of restaurant lunches, snack machines and desks full of candy and other snacks. It offers you a unique opportunity to start on the path toward transforming your diet lifestyle.

Your quest for significant behavior change deserves your undivided attention, at least in the beginning. A successful launch of your dietary lifestyle transformation program gives you solid motivation to continue your efforts for a substantial time going forward.

The night before your chosen start date, have a pre-celebratory dinner with your significant other and/or close friends. It serves as a symbolic kickoff event for your journey to achieving the change(s) you desire in your weight and your life as well as a signal to yourself and others of your serious intent to make changes in your life. While I do not recommend a blowout, super-high-calorie, high-alcohol event, a dinner and social occasion is appropriate and desirable.

Prior to your start date, have a preparation period, perhaps a week ahead. First, prepare your mind for the challenge ahead. Review your reasons for wanting to lose weight and change your diet lifestyle and alert your partner, friends and colleagues of your goals. Also, strive to prep your mind to be maximally receptive to new suggestions and new routines. Two excellent ways to do this are to engage in increased physical activity and to be more rested by sleeping longer.

Preparing Your Environment

Prepare your physical environment, home, office, and maybe car for some of you, to support your goals. Specifically, you should make a sweep of your home and office to remove the most readily accessible sources of high-sugar, high-simple carb, empty calorie snacks, or at least move them to a much less visible and harder-to-reach location.

In addition, it is wise to stock your home and office with healthful foods and snacks. All of us have certain meals that are more problematic than others. For some, it might be a rushed breakfast heading out the door. For others, it might be the accessibility of fast food restaurants at work. It's a great idea to prepare healthful meals in advance for problematic times and make your journey easier.

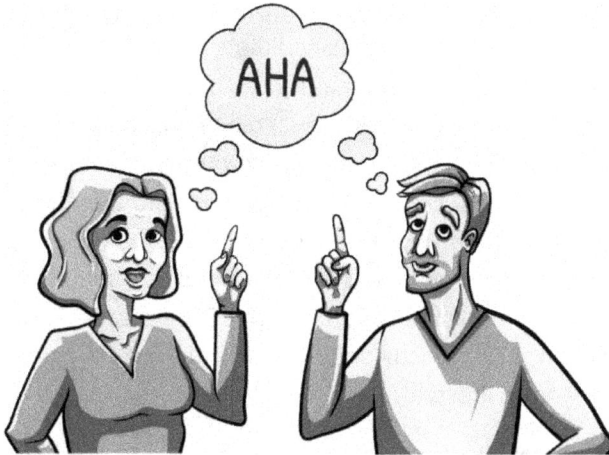

- Weight loss is difficult, as the urge to overeat is an instinct bred into your DNA, but it does not have to be your destiny. Instincts do drive your behavior, but they are tendencies, not certainties.
- Only real lifestyle change can lead to successful long-term weight loss, and to achieve this goal, automatic, negative responses must be replaced with positive, healthy habits. This is not the goal of traditional temporary diets, nor can they do this. Starting one more traditional diet, and expecting a different outcome, is truly the triumph of hope over experience. Remember, Albert Einstein's definition of irrationality is doing the same thing over and over and expecting to get a different outcome. Approach your dietary lifestyle program as if your life depends on it, because it does!

Chapter 4: How and Why the Whole Brain Diet Lifestyle Works

Extrinsic incentives may get you going, but it's intrinsic factors that sustain your motivation over the long-run.

Why Diets Fail

To understand why the Whole Brain Diet Lifestyle plan works, we must first review why alternative diet lifestyles and diets do not work. For most of us, when we say we are on a diet, it means a temporary change from our normal, typical behavior. When we, if we, reach our weight loss goal, we typically revert back to our more customary routines. Diets are not sustainable long-term. First, we never learn how to fundamentally change our behavior and our habits. Second, weight loss is the avowed goal, once reached, we feel that the mission is accomplished and abandon the behaviors that led to the initial loss in weight. Diets place an inappropriate and ineffective emphasis strictly on losing pounds, not changing or creating, a healthier, long-term lifestyle.

At a more basic level, diets are not effective in the long term because the motivation and incentive to lose weight is based mostly on "extrinsic" factors. Aside from potential health concerns, most of us want to lose weight to make ourselves more appealing to others. If we reach our desired weight loss, the goal is achieved. The motivation for continuing deprivation (what most diets are really about) ceases to be as relevant and the weight is slowly regained. Additionally, your body fights back against your weight loss to undermine you and make sustaining a loss much more difficult.

How is the Whole Brain Diet Lifestyle plan different? At its core, the Whole Brain Diet Lifestyle plan is about changing your behavior and instilling new habits that naturally lead to a healthier life, resulting in better well-being. Fundamentally, the plan focuses on behavior and habit creation, not the number of pounds lost. If you successfully adopt and sustain the Whole Brain Diet Lifestyle plan and enter a weightless state of being, weight loss occurs as a byproduct of the process, not the primary goal.

New Theory of Intrinsic Motivation

Of course, these benefits are contingent on adopting and following the Whole Brain Diet Lifestyle plan. This plan is more sustainable than a traditional diet or other lifestyles. It is based on the Self-Determination Theory (SDT for short) described in Daniel Pink's book, *Drive*.[1] This theory states that we are all subject to universal and fundamental psychological needs. SDT identify three that are especially powerful as a basis for sustained motivation. These needs are the innate desire for autonomy, competence and connectedness.[2]

In the past, psychologists identified only two basic drives fundamental to human beings:

- The primal biological drives to satisfy our hunger, thirst and our desire/need for sex.
- The drive to seek rewards/pleasure and avoid penalties/pain.

Professors Deci and Ryan identified a third drive based on innate psychological needs, which supplements and complements the first two. They point out that for optimal performance in some activities, the desire to receive rewards and avoid punishment is primary and highly effective as a motivator. But it is only ideal for the most rote and least challenging parts of our work and of our life. Extrinsic rewards or punishments fail to be a very effective motivator for more creative and complex activities. For this, intrinsic rewards are most effective and retain their effectiveness repeatedly over the long-run.

How the Intrinsic Motivation Theory is Consistent with the Whole Brain Diet Lifestyle plan

The Whole Brain Diet Lifestyle plan is consistent with the intrinsic motivation theory, as it is designed to deliver a whole way of life, not a single, quantifiable goal (such as the number of pounds lost). The benefits you get from following this lifestyle change your life in ways that are not always easily quantified, but are obvious when realized. As it relates to Deci and Ryan's SDT theory, the Whole Brain Diet Lifestyle plan offers the following intrinsic benefits:

- Autonomy and self-directedness (you decide how, when and how quickly to proceed)
- Personal choice (you have many choices to choose from)
- Support via social connectedness (you are encouraged to make your quest for transformation known to others and even better to share your quest with a partner or friend)

- A path for ever-increasing mastery (you can continue to get better and better at living the Whole Brain Diet Lifestyle without limits)
- A challenge that stretches you, but is perceived as doable (the multiplicity of tactics you can choose from, makes the plan seem doable)

With this plan, you can choose to construct three broadly different strategic barriers (or all three) that are based on restricting ready access to high-sugar, high simple-carb, high-calorie foods using:

Psychological barriers: Chapter 9
Social barriers: Chapter 10
Physical barriers: Chapter 11

Within each of these strategic paths are multiple tactics you can adopt to best serve your individual needs and your individual preferences.

There is no specific endpoint, no final level of lifestyle perfection. Therefore, the pursuit of competence, of ever-increasing mastery, continues to be present indefinitely as a motivating force (and the desire for mastery is one of the innate drives we human beings possess). You can follow the Whole Brain Diet Lifestyle plan like playing a game, where simply playing the game is the reward itself. Over the long-run as you follow the Whole Brain Diet Lifestyle, you receive feedback from your mind and from your body that is rewarding because it makes you feel good. We are all inclined to continue to engage in behaviors that make us feel good.

Implementing and sustaining the Whole Brain Diet Lifestyle is highly compatible with the SDT theory and continually offers you intrinsic rewards to motivate you for a lifetime and keep you moving on the path toward a weightless state of being.

Why the Whole Brain Diet Lifestyle Plan Will Work for You?
The core reason why the plan will actually work for you and how the plan helps you to change your behavior and instill new, healthy habits is simply mindfulness.

One definition of mindfulness is, "a mental state achieved by focusing one's awareness on the present moment, while calmly acknowledging and accepting one's feelings, thoughts and bodily sensations."[3] The key is that when you are mindful, you are focused intently on the present moment. ***The easiest and best method I have found to instantly become mindful is to use the Take 5 technique.*** Once you invoke it, you immediately become more mindful of the emotional cravings you are experiencing that drive you to snack unhealthfully and to overeat, and hence you are better able to defuse these cravings.

In recent years, mindfulness has become a very trendy word in our lexicon. It has been trumpeted as the answer to solving many problems, to facing many personal challenges. It may seem unbelievable, but it is real, it is powerful, and its use can be transformational. Holocaust survivor and philosopher Viktor Frankl summed up the essence of mindfulness when he said, "Between stimulus and response there is a space. In the space is our power to choose a response. In our response lies our growth and freedom." We all have the power to choose.

When you are truly mindful, each discrete moment is distinguishable. You are able to be present in the moment, for each and every moment. You have time to react, to make a deliberate decision. You have time to either give in to a fleeting craving or to allow it to dissipate without controlling your behavior. Being mindful gives you the illusion of time standing still. You become momentarily detached from the impulses that drive poor judgement. It gives you the ability to make the choice to follow your *Skinny* brain, not your *Fat* brain.

Provocative recent research conducted by Eric Robinson of the University of Liverpool gives strong, additional credibility to the importance of eating with a mindful awareness. His research indicates there is a relationship between being obese and one's cognitive function, including one's memory. Being obese degrades your memory of events and activities, meaning obese people have a less vivid, less powerful memory of their eating experiences. Robinson said, "Our research suggests that you might eat more if you have an impaired memory, so you end up in a vicious cycle where memory's impaired by an unhealthy lifestyle and then that impairment promotes over-consumption."[4]

This hypothesis gained some traction in additional research Robinson conducted. This research showed when he created a higher level of awareness, hence memory, of a meal in people's minds, they ate less at the next food consumption occasion.

One not too difficult way to increase your awareness of what you ate is to jot it down and enter each food item into a food journal or directly into your smartphone. Before your next meal, review what you consumed at your last meal. As Eric Robinson's research suggests, the more top-of-mind is your awareness of what you last ate, the more you think about and pay attention to what you choose to eat at the next meal occasion. This makes you more mindful of your food choices and subsequently impacts how much you actually choose to eat. This simple action can result in fewer total calories being consumed.

An important part of this book is to create an awareness and understanding of the environmental or situational factors that generate the cues that trigger your cravings. Once you have this understanding, you can combine it with the ability to deter a craving impulse by using the Take 5 technique. Over time, along with your intention to be mindful, you create a state of consciousness that connects you to each moment, allowing you to make a deliberate choice on how you want to proceed.

I will show you many ways to enhance and maintain your mental energy. When you have more mental energy and you continually receive the intrinsic rewards provided by following the Whole Brain Diet Lifestyle plan, creating new behavioral responses and new routines is far easier to accomplish. These new patterns of behavioral responses become second nature, they become habitual and a healthier lifestyle is the long-run result. Entering a weightless state of being becomes a reality.

Recent research reviewed a large number of brain imaging studies and concluded that there may be a common neural basis for cravings, including cravings for gambling, sex, drugs and food.[5] The brain areas responsible for forming habits and for self-control act to make such cravings be virtually irresistible to some people and influential for all of us. This study also makes clear that your environment – psychological and physical – has a great impact on your ability to deter a craving. It makes sense to change your environment if you want to change your life and your lifestyle.

Being highly mindful is one of the best ways to live in the moment and allow yourself a brief, but real opportunity to give in to a craving or to allow it to simply fade away. Mindfulness is the secret path to changing your dietary lifestyle and explains why the Whole Brain Diet Lifestyle plan works. Using the Take 5 technique is a highly effective and rapid means to reach a more mindful state of being.

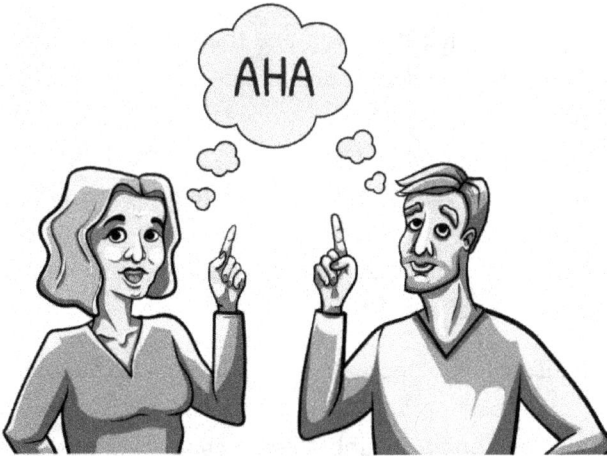

- Weight loss is a natural byproduct of following the Whole Brain Diet Lifestyle, not its only goal, but by following the plan weight loss occurs.
- Mindfulness is a "new-agey" catch phrase, but it is very real, and its benefits are very powerful and practicing it can transform your life.

Chapter 5: The Concept and Role of Mental Energy

Many people may not be able to define it, but they always know when they have it and when they do not.

What is Mental Energy?

Mental energy is a psychic state or mood that provides a force to direct your mind and/or your behavior toward a desired pursuit or goal.[1] When you are mentally energized, you have more will and resolve to engage in activities that you choose to pursue. When your mental energy is low or depleted, you are less focused and less motivated toward accomplishing a desired goal and more likely to be distracted from this pursuit. Mental energy is the stuff that fuels your willpower and resolve and supports the maintenance of your self-control.

Mental energy is a bit analogous to what Supreme Court Justice Potter Stewart said about pornography, "I can't define it, but I know it when I see it." You may not personally be able to easily and readily define mental energy, but you know when you have it and when you don't. When you have it, your mind is alert and sharp, and you are able to follow through on the activities that you focus on. When you do not have it, your mind is distracted, unfocused and less purposeful. I think everyone can relate to and intuitively understand this state of mind.

When you are able to maximize and sustain your mental energy, you can also maximize and sustain your level of self-control. You can use this self-control to instill new healthy behaviors long enough for them to become internalized and routine. Once this happens, you achieve the long-term behavioral changes you seek, which makes your life healthier, happier and more productive.

The ultimate question becomes: What can be done to build and sustain your mental energy long enough to cover the transitional period (often at least eight to sixteen weeks), needed to activate the new behavioral responses and habits that you seek to establish?[2] Of course you should be aware that very small changes to behavior may take less time to establish, while highly significant and major deviations from old routines may take longer.

How to Sustain and Build Mental Energy

Few of us have a natural, sustained level of mental energy high enough to carry us through the transitional period where new habits and routines are formed and become ingrained.

There are two strategic approaches to follow to maintain and build your mental energy: sustaining and maximizing. Sustaining refers to actions taken to minimize the depletion or use of your mental energy and therefore help keep it at a high enough level to be productive. Maximizing refers to actions taken that actually increase or boost your mental energy.

Sustaining strategies include behaviors in the following areas:

- Using the Take 5 technique
- Striving to adopt and follow a *Lite* approach to life which is explained in the following chapter
- Psychological/social/physical barriers to high-sugar, high-carb, high-calorie snacks/foods
- Use of highly scheduled and pre-planned life activities
- Tactics to limit decision making and minimize free choice

Using the Take 5 technique is one of the best and easiest ways to help sustain your mental energy. Trying to rely on sheer force of will to abstain from eating a high-sugar, high-calorie snack is very mental-energy depleting. Take 5 lets you rely on a brief pause in time and on your physical energy when you remove yourself from the location where your craving originated and from where the actual sugary snacks are typically stored so that you can be more mindful. Using Take 5, you do not have to rely solely on your willpower alone.

Maximizing strategies include behaviors in the following areas:

- Use of memes
- Employ the principles of embodied cognition (Chapter 17)
- Exercise and physical activity
- Stress management and stress reduction
- Sleep practices and good sleep hygiene
- Creation and expression of compassion
- Reading positive psychological statements and viewing positive visual images

Dieting and Self-Control

Dieting and weight loss create a highly difficult test of self-control. You start each day with good intentions, but each act of resistance or denial lowers your subsequent willpower and resolve. As willpower weakens, you need to renew or replenish it. Many researchers believe that the fastest and most reliable means to boost your willpower is to ingest sugary foods, which quickly convert to glucose to instantly fuel the body and elevate (at least temporarily) the spirit.[3] However, this reinforces the very behavior you are trying to minimize. A better alternative is to increase your willpower by non-food means and/or to avoid or minimize the situations in which your willpower is depleted by your resisting temptations to consume unhealthy foods or snacks.

Remember that your brain loves constancy, familiarity and routine but places no value judgment on the positivity or negativity of such behaviors. These states make your brain happy, and a happy brain is motivated to continue those behaviors and routines. Once established, whether positive or negative, healthy or unhealthy, the brain is attuned to continue those behaviors. If you can find a means to persevere long enough for old, unhealthy behaviors to be replaced by newer, healthier ones, you realize long-term, transformational change to your diet lifestyle and to your life.

As you progress through each of the subsequent chapters, you are able to see how these sustaining and maximizing strategies complement each other to facilitate and promote the transformational changes to your diet lifestyle that you are seeking. Taken together, these strategies and tools greatly increase the likelihood that significant behavioral changes occur and last over the long-run.

Even after you establish new patterns of behavior, some of the old cues that triggered previously unhealthful food responses can re-emerge. You may succumb to temptations and fall back into old, unwanted behaviors. So, it is best to continue to keep in place the same psychological, social and physical barriers to food accessibility. These barriers reinforce your mental energy, willpower and self-control into the future, well past the initial establishment of new routines. If you reach a true state of weightlessness, then you need much less vigilance as your conscious and unconscious mind are united to support your new healthier lifestyle.

Mental energy is the independent facilitating factor that makes the process work. Create more mental energy, and you automatically fuel your willpower and self-control, making long-term behavioral change possible. Mental energy is the key.

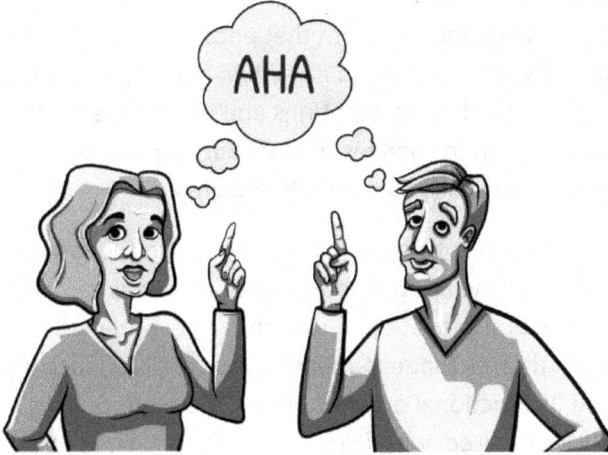

- The creation and maintenance of mental energy is a vital, facilitating factor in achieving your goal of making long-term transformational changes to your dietary behavior. Behavioral change is the goal, and mental energy is the fuel that drives the process.

- Mental energy supports your willpower and self-control. While it is easily depleted, it can also be readily renewed, and there are many alternative means available to accomplish this.

Chapter 6: Neuroplasticity and Behavior Change

The neurons that fire together, wire together, and as a result new habitual behaviors are created.

What Is Neuroplasticity?

Neuroplasticity is an umbrella term that encompasses synaptic and non-synaptic plasticity, i.e., it refers to growth in neural pathways that are due to changes in one's behavior, emotions and environment.[1] Research indicates that your brain changes throughout your life, and we as individuals have the ability to direct their course.

Research shows that "substantial change occurs in the lowest neocortical processing areas of the brain, and that these changes can profoundly alter the pattern of neural activation in response to experience. Neuroscience research also indicates that experience can actually change both the brain's structure and its functional organization."[2] The adult brain is not permanently hard-wired, with fixed neuronal circuits. In response to training and experience, it can be rewired to result in changes in your responses to stimuli. This way, old, automatic behaviors rooted in your reptilian brain can be countered with new, healthier alternatives desired by your conscious, higher-order brain (i.e., the neocortex). While the path of least resistance is to respond habitually, your old habits can be overridden and supplanted by new habits. The more entrenched a habit is, the more resistant it is to change. But through perseverance and repetition of new thoughts, emotions and behaviors, these habits can be altered.[3]

How to Promote Neurogenesis

Some of the most important ways to promote neurogenesis and build new neuronal connections and interconnections are by:[4]

- Using the Take 5 technique.
- Exercising, which builds body and brain fitness.
- Practicing meditation.
- Engaging in new life experiences, activities and events.
- Learning how to do familiar tasks differently.
- Managing and reducing stress, which is incompatible with neuronal growth and neurogenesis.
- Being more engaged, focused, and alert.
- Welcoming unexpected and surprise events.

- Continually working toward achieving high and higher levels of mastery in the skills you seek.
- Remembering that the more powerful and vivid the emotional context of any experience, the more powerful the association and the more robust the accompanying neurogenic growth.
- Practicing a "lite" mind-set and a lite way of life that makes the brain happy.
- Making new friends and staying socially connected.
- Being mindful of everything you do, see, feel and experience as this contributes to neuronal growth.
- Seeking to continually enrich your life in small and large ways.

Generally speaking, you can choose to construct your life and your environment to naturally promote brain fitness and growth via neurogenesis. All of your experiences and all of your behaviors impact neuron development. Positive behaviors promote neuron growth, and negative behaviors (like excessive alcohol consumption, acute stress or a highly sedentary lifestyle) promote neuronal death.

Take 5 is a positive behavior that drives neuron growth as it helps to train your brain to abstain from instantly yielding to a craving to eat a high-sugar snack. By repetitively practicing Take 5, neurons that promote taking a pause to interrupt your emotional craving impulses are strengthened and become more likely to be activated again in similar circumstances.

How Neurogenesis Contributes to Behavioral Transformation

Increasing brain health and fitness via neurogenesis is a critical factor that results in forming new habitual responses. By creating and using your mental energy, you move this process forward to a successful conclusion. Your mental energy provides the power that allows you to persevere and repeat the new behavioral routines you wish to establish long enough for them to take root and become internalized. In this way, the neurons in your brain become wired together, and new habits are created.

Once your routines become automatic, you have less need to be continually mindful, alert and vigilant to temptations to unhealthful foods. You become less subject to the cravings that precipitate their consumption and more able to deflect the cravings that you do experience. While you never completely extinguish the cravings for sugar and fat and the instinct to overeat, you are in a position to manage them and to counter their negative effects. With effort you can silence (or at least quiet) a million years of evolutionary instincts that drive overeating and obesity.

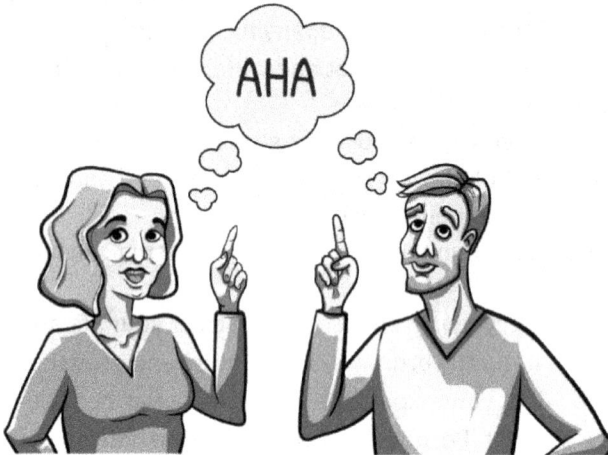

- Neurogenesis sounds complicated, but it is not. Many activities based on your thoughts, emotions and behaviors that are healthy for your body are also healthy for your brain. Repetition of these activities enrich and expand your brain's neural network, thereby promoting behavioral change.
- You naturally choose to repeat activities that reward your brain and make it happy. But your brain does not place a value judgment on the positivity or negativity of these behaviors. You must possess enough self-awareness to distance yourself from these behaviors and assess how healthy they really are for you. Even if you are not very self-aware now, you can nurture this quality and increase it with conscious and repetitive effort.

Chapter 7: A *"Lite"* Approach to Life

Lightness may describe one's weight, but "liteness" describes a basic approach to living your life.

One conscious, deliberate action that you can take is adopting and following a lite approach to life. In early humans, a "heavy" lifestyle, focusing on existential threats to one's existence, was life-affirming and protective of self-preservation. Today this orientation runs counter to its original purpose by directing us to eat heavy – to eat a large quantity of high-simple-carb, high-sugar foods. Use conscious intent to adopt a lite approach to life as your customary lifestyle; a life that is lite in mind-set, mood and food consumption. Striving for a lite approach to life is an important part of realizing your ambition to achieve a diet lifestyle transformation.

What does it mean to live lite? Let's start with a dictionary definition of the word "lightness":

- The state or quality of having little weight or force
- Ease of quickness of movement; agility
- Ease or cheerfulness in manner or style
- Freedom from worry or trouble
- Lack of appropriate seriousness; levity
- Delicacy or subtlety in craft, performance, or effect[1]

My take on creating a "lite" approach to life includes the following:

- Seeking liteness of spirit
- Seeking liteness of mood
- Seeking liteness in foods/snacks
- Seeking liteness to illuminate your negative, automatic thinking patterns; to uncover and expose your habitual, heavy behaviors

A lite lifestyle promotes a happy brain because liteness feels good, and your brain likes to feel good. These good feelings naturally help to fuel and sustain your mental energy, which is drained by heavy, negative mood states and thinking patterns. Liteness is restorative, rejuvenating to yourself, while a heavy approach to life saps energy, depleting your willpower and undermining your self-control. When you live a lite lifestyle, it ushers you into a weightless state of being. While being lite and weightless are not the same thing, they are entirely compatible and complementary to one another. A liteness of being has implications for your:

- Psychological state of mind
- Social relationships and interactions
- Behaviors related to food purchase and consumption, exercise, stress mitigation and compassionate intent

A Lite Versus Heavy Lifestyle

You can make a deliberate, conscious choice to go lite or go heavy in your thinking and behaviors. Going lite makes you more agile, more adaptive, and more flexible in your responses and your behaviors, while going heavy ties you into repeating the same non-adaptive automatic, negative behaviors that play a large part in most of our lives. Sometimes going heavy is appropriate and life-affirming. When facing an immediate threat to your life, you want your instincts to kick in and activate a fight-or-flight response. There are times when you may consciously, by your own volition, choose to engage in heavy thoughts, feelings, conversations, and / or heavy foods. But this should be limited and on your own terms, not driven by the whims of your subconscious emotions. If your normal default mode is one of liteness, you are likely to be happier, more dynamic and more adaptive. These states, by supporting your mental energy, make achieving transformational change much more likely.

A Call to Action: The Take 5 Mantra

Striving for liteness is more than a philosophy of living; it is a specific call to action. When you are faced with an immediate urge or craving to snack at an unplanned time, you should enlist the following mental aid. Visualize yourself locked in a struggle between your *Fat* brain and your *Skinny* brain, between liteness and heaviness, and repeat the following mantra, by literally telling yourself to "Take 5 - Take 5, Take 5 – (*Your Name*) chooses to follow his/her *Skinny* brain!" This mental refrain instantly spikes your mental energy and liteness boosting your willpower and enhancing your self-control. Sticking to a lite approach to life helps you follow your *Skinny* brain and allows an immediate craving to dissipate.

The Take 5 mantra encapsulates much of what you will learn about behavioral transformation tools and tactics in the chapters that follow. You have the ability to summon this advice instantaneously by repeating the Take 5 mantra. By understanding that your brain is the master of your behavior and that YOU are the master of your brain, you will know that for any immediate food consumption choice you are facing, the power to resist it is a choice you can consciously make. Take 5 helps you to "be the user of our brain, not simply be used by it," as Tanzi and Chopra postulate in their book *Super Brain*.

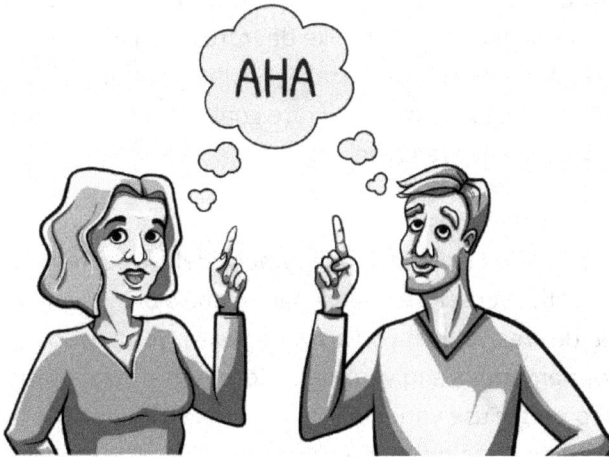

- Emotions and behaviors are contagious; they are like infectious viruses that can spread from one person to another. If you want to adopt a lite approach to life that supports your mental energy and promotes weight loss, you should strive to incorporate a liteness of being and to associate with people who themselves are lite in spirit and in weight.
- You can most effectively break a craving in the instant when you first feel it. Use the Take 5 mantra as an emotional circuit breaker to allow a craving to dissipate and float harmlessly away. You should literally have an internal debate with yourself, which allows you to make a conscious choice to go lite and forgo an unhealthful snack at the point of maximum vulnerability, i.e., the moment you experience a craving.

Chapter 8: Setting New Goals and Creating New Habits

Your intentions spur you to create goals, your habitual behaviors make them happen or not.

There are many books devoted to offering advice on how to set goals and how to achieve them. Too many of us live our lives like we're a pinball careening from one bumper event to another with no control over where we are headed. While others are like deer frozen in a headlight, unable to move, too fearful of making a mistake. Having positive habits help you to overcome these obstacles and facilitate goal achievement by purposeful action not just reflexive reaction.

What Is Self-Awareness

Self-awareness is an important topic. One widely accepted definition of awareness is, "the conscious knowledge of one's own character, feelings, motives and desires.[1] When you are self-aware, you are able to observe yourself, your emotions and your behaviors with some detachment. This allows you to better use your conscious intent to guide your behavior rather than being ruled by your automatic, habitual responses. Letting go is a path to self-awareness.

It follows that the more self-aware you are, the better you know yourself. Being more self-aware is the trait that shapes your intentions, which you create to provide vital input for the goals you want to achieve.

Beyond this, self-awareness also boosts or hinders realizing your goals. When you are highly self-aware, you more readily identify the personal and environmental obstacles that may get in the way of achieving your goals. On many levels being more self-aware lays down a path for you to follow that is less conflicted and more purposefully compatible with your true nature. This makes achieving your goals much more likely.

Being more self-aware gives you the capacity to recognize the cues and trigger points that move you further away from goal attainment. It also helps you to counter these tendencies before they impact your behavior.

Two of the best activities are exercise and meditation. These activities put you in touch with your body and your mind, heightening your sense of separation from others and your environment. Both of these are central to the plan to transform your diet lifestyle. When you follow this plan, you naturally and automatically increase your self-awareness, and this self-awareness helps to make the plan more likely to work for you.

A valid question to ask yourself is, can you become too self-aware, i.e., obsessively aware? Being obsessive about some aspects of your behavior is not necessarily a bad thing. In this context, by obsessive I mean that you are hyper-vigilant about your eating environment, what you eat, when you eat and how much you eat until your diet lifestyle is where you want it to be and you have entered a weightless state of being.

When your diet lifestyle improves, you will most likely no longer be obese, and that is equivalent health-wise to moving away from an existential danger to your life. You can reduce your likelihood of having a heart attack, a stroke or even cancer to a nearly normal level. Along with this, there are very real psychosocial benefits that go along with significantly improving your lifestyle and reducing your weight. Extremism in the defense of your health, well-being and longevity is justifiable and may be needed to accomplish your goals.

If, like a former smoker or heavy drinker, you followed an unhealthy lifestyle and were once obese, you will always have a risk of relapse unless you truly reach a weightless state of being. Unlike a smoker or problem drinker, one high-sugar, high-calorie snack is not likely to cause you to abandon your striving to transform your diet lifestyle. But you must be highly self-aware and mindful to avoid falling back into patterns that leads to a lifestyle relapse and an inevitable weight gain. If this requires some degree of obsessiveness, then the end will more than justify the means.

Nurturing your self-awareness and becoming more self-aware are the keys to maximizing the likelihood you achieve real and lasting dietary lifestyle transformation. As Shakespeare said in his most iconic play, *Hamlet*, "To thine own self be true." If you do not do this, making your goals a reality is far more difficult.

Use of a Reward and Penalty Program
Another very viable means to effect change and realize your ultimate lifestyle goal is to structure a reward and penalty program commensurate with the importance and magnitude of the changes you are seeking.[2] To do

this you should set up, in advance, a series of rewards you receive when you reach certain, specific behavioral milestones. While a milestone might be measured in pounds lost, it could also be dropping a pant or dress size or the ability to walk an additional mile. Additionally, to complement the positive, it also makes sense to build in some disincentives when you fail to reach your milestone(s) in a timely and prescribed fashion. Using a series of rewards and penalties can be a highly useful means to supplement the intrinsic motivations that are an integral part of the Whole Brain Diet Lifestyle.

Rewards may be anything of value to you, except they should not involve food. You may find rewards that involve doing and experiencing things as more motivating and appreciated longer than physical objects.[3] Your particular choice can be left to your own determination. If you intend to try and effect change over a one-year period, then create a series of rewards to mirror various time periods that expire over that one-year time frame.

Research suggests that a series of small, frequent rewards can have a very consequential impact on your behavior. Plan a weekly or bi-weekly reward for successfully following the Whole Brain Diet Lifestyle. You might treat yourself to a movie outing or some other small reward. In the age of the Coronavirus, it might not be a physical outing, but renting a movie or making a small purchase. At the end of each month and quarter, select a progressively larger and more important reward commensurate with how well you are moving toward your ultimate lifestyle goals. At the end of the year, if you have successfully altered your lifestyle a large and significant reward is justified. Research suggests that even more compelling than giving yourself a reward is to share it with a significant other or even give it to him or her exclusively. There is truth to the saying that it is better to give then to receive.

One means you can use to implement the large end-of-year reward involves putting a pre-set sum of money aside at the beginning of your journey toward your ultimate goal. This money can be used either as a reward or as a penalty if you fail to meet your final objective.[4] You could deposit this sum of money in a one-year CD that is difficult to tap into or remove. If you successfully meet your goal, use the money to purchase your reward.

If you do not meet your goal, an excellent tactic is to give it away to a charity that you would typically not choose to support. Even better, commit to donating the money to a cause which you do not agree with, and this may increase your motivation to fulfill your lifestyle goals even more.

Research shows that the use of such positive incentives, coupled with a potential negative incentive, can be quite consequential in facilitating change. The financial reward or penalty you employ should be large enough to be truly significant to you for optimum, motivational effect.

In order for this reward/penalty process to be most effective the following conditions should be met.[5]

- The reward must be directly associated with achieving a behavioral milestone.
- The timing of the reward should be very close to the attainment of the milestone you are seeking.
- The reward/penalty must be consequential enough to make a difference to you.
- You must believe that the reward/penalty will actually occur as planned.
- The reward/penalty process is often best if administered or overseen by an objective third party who can assure that the appropriate incentive or disincentive is meted out.

Using a reward program allows you to utilize an external source of willpower instead of relying solely on your internal willpower and resolve. Using this tactic helps to boost your mental energy and hence your self-control.

Instead of putting obstacles to success in your path, the real objective is to put in place a structure that nudges you in the direction of the kind of changes in behavior that you are hoping to realize.[6]

Kelly Traver framed it nicely in her book *The Program: The Brain-Smart Approach to the Healthiest You* when she encouraged us not to underestimate the power of your immediate environment on your behavior. She continued by saying that you should set up the world around you, as much as you can, to trigger your brain toward healthy behavior.[7]

Translating an Intention into a Habitual Behavior

As Tanzi and Chopra state in their book *Super Brain,* thoughts are not actions, just fleeting mental images. Thoughts have no consequences until you choose to make them important.[7] Waldman and Newberg also said that intent drives our focus, and when it is clearly stated and repetitively reinforced, it engages the brain to facilitate and promote the goals of our intent.[9]

An outline of the change process shows the following:[9]

- It starts with a feeling that bubbles up from your emotional subconscious.
- This feeling is brought to your consciousness as a thought.
- The thought morphs into an intention to do something.
- You start to act on the intention voluntarily and deliberately.
- You repeat and practice the behavior(s) that you want to become permanent.
- The repetition of the mental and physical changes starts to infuse your subconscious.
- Your subconscious aligns with your conscious self to reinforce the behavioral changes.
- The intended changes become internalized, and old, unwanted automatic behaviors are supplanted with new behavioral response patterns.
- The new behavior(s) become routine and habitual.

Following these steps, you circumvent your old behavioral responses and instill new behavioral patterns in their place. It is vital to understand and accept that the brain is naturally resistant to change; it wants stability and predictability. As such, it is crucial to try and counter your brain's natural instinct to resist change by making small, gradual changes to your behavior, giving your brain time to adjust to a new reality.[10]

Are Weight Loss Goals Necessary

It is OK, even laudable, to have some grand, high-level goals to the end game associated with making a fundamental change to your lifestyle. These may include worthy goals such as losing weight (even very large weight losses), increasing your energy level, eating a more nutritionally balanced and healthful diet, reducing stress, and leading an overall happier life.

Although I do not recommend setting a specific weight loss goal, there is some research that suggests that if weight loss is part of your plan in adopting a better and healthier lifestyle, then having a weight loss goal that is very challenging may result in a greater weight loss than a more modest goal.[11] While it is better to not have a specific weight loss goal in terms of number of pounds you want to lose, you want a goal that can be quantified. For example, a person might set their aspirational goal to "lose" "X" number of dress or pant sizes (e.g., 3 to 4).

The secret is planning to get there in small, very finite steps to give your body and your brain time to adjust and minimize their natural resistance to major deviations from your routine and from a large, rapid weight loss. Trying to quickly make large and dramatic changes greatly depletes your mental energy, whereas making smaller, more gradual changes helps to conserve it. Goals of this fashion gives you built-in milestones to mark your progress. If you adopt and consistently follow the Whole Brain Diet Lifestyle, you will lose weight. I suggest tracking your weight loss as an indicator of how well you are doing in changing your diet lifestyle. While weight loss is only one possible indicator, it is, for most of us who are overweight, an important one.

When your weight stabilizes at a level that feels right for your body and your mind, you have lost enough weight. By this time, for most of you, you will have lost enough weight to be noticeable and you will have succeeded in making your appearance more appealing to others. Your diet becomes much more healthful as well. Aren't these the things that make losing weight worthwhile?

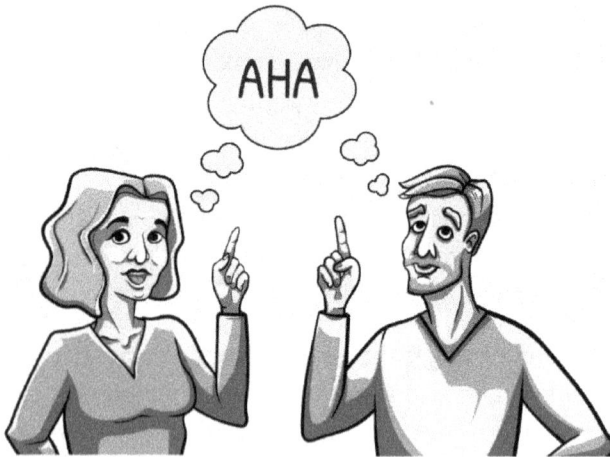

- If you do not know where you want to go with your life, it is not likely you will achieve what you want or what you are capable of achieving. Setting goals, even if life gets in the way, lays down a path to help you reach your potential.
- By creating more positive, more productive habits, you reduce a drain on your mental energy that frequent decision-making creates. Relying on habitual behaviors simplifies your life and thereby promotes goal achievement.

Part 3:

Maintaining and Building Mental Energy

Chapter 9: Psychological Barriers
Always remember, "Your brain is the master of your behavior and YOU are the master of your brain."

Psychological Principles
Mental techniques are an important and integral part of the Whole Brain Diet Lifestyle plan. Psychological principles are one of the pillars on which this lifestyle is built. Let's begin by reviewing some background, principles and theories upon which this plan is based.

Your Brain Is Out-Of-Sync with the Modern World
Our brains evolved over many millennia to ensure our preservation and survival.[1] Primitive hominid species were in existence, and before this, the kernel of our humanity was encapsulated in the bodies and minds of the great apes and chimpanzees. Our brains and our genetic heritage evolved when the pace of change in the environment was very, very slow. Highly significant evolutionary changes were manifested only over many thousands of generations. Our brains, often untrained, unaware and instinctually driven, are no match for the new ever present availability of abundant food, especially high-sugar, ultra-processed foods.[2]

Employing the Take 5 technique mitigates this pervasive cue with an equally accessible countermeasure. Wherever you are, whatever you are doing, use a Take 5 pause to interrupt an impulse to eat. Simply thinking to yourself "Take 5" is enough, with practice, to automatically activate the Take 5 response. Take 5 gives you time to re-sync your intention to eat smart – eat in moderation with your conscious, purposeful brain so that you always have a choice to yield to a craving or not. The Take 5 technique readily counters the ever present access to food that so many of us have in this era of the Coronavirus.

Our instincts do drive much of our behavior. In the book *Super Genes*, Rudy Tanzi and Deepak Chopra weigh in on this matter when they say that although hard-wired in our brain instincts are tendencies, they are not our destiny. Our conscious mind can override and redirect these tendencies.[3] This is fundamental to your understanding and accepting that a transformational change in your lifestyle is possible.

The Brain: A Primer

In *Virus of the Mind*, Richard Brodie states the purpose of our brain and why it evolved is to increase our chance of surviving to the age of reproduction and beyond, to increase the number of children we produce and to increase our chance to mate with a high-quality partner. These primal goals drive much, or even all our behavior.

The brain evolved into three basic parts. The first and most ancient part is the reptilian brain, including our brain stem.[4] This part of our brain controls and regulates our most basic bodily functions and is embedded in a deeply subconscious part of our reality. We cannot see into this part of our brain, and we have little ability to control or effect what transpires there. The functions controlled by our reptilian brain are automatic and fundamental to our survival.

The next layer of our brain is called the limbic system. It houses our emotional circuitry. This is the part of the brain that we typically refer to as our subconscious.[5] It is also the part of our brain most responsible for the decision-making process guided by the impulses and thoughts that bubble up from our subconscious. Many believe that most of what we describe as thinking is really the result of our subconscious.[6] This does not mean, nor is it intended to imply, that we are irrational or non-deliberative beings who respond only to our emotions. But it does mean that many of the reasons we ascribe to the decisions that we have made are often rationalizations for the choices that are deeply influenced and directed by our subconscious.[7]

Our brain and our subconscious crave predictability, stability and routine, and this is why we so stubbornly cling to our habitual, automatic behaviors.[8] Our instincts and our ancient drives created neural pathways in our brains that are deeply rooted and hard to resist. However, this is absolutely key, these pathways can be altered via neurogenesis, in which new neural connections are made. These pathways provide the impetus for you to adhere to your routines and habits but can be modified by using your rational, deliberate brain guided by your intention to alter your behavior.[9]

Our brains are the ultimate arbiter of our decision-making and the driver of our behavior. As such, we need to look inside ourselves as a starting point to creating an environment for ourselves where food is less accessible. First, how does your psychological state make food more or less desirable and accessible? Second, how can you use your brain to counteract the ancient drives, which when combined with your ever-present accessibility to food, promote overeating, bingeing and inappropriate snacking?

Creating New Automatic Behaviors

It takes considerable work and time to alter your habitual responses. Just as it takes time to create a new path through a woods or meadow, you must reinforce your behavior many times to create a new path for your behavioral responses.[10] To counter old, automatic behaviors with new response patterns, you must have a real intent and the will to repeat the new pattern many times until it becomes routine. You need considerable time to allow your brain to follow your intentions to internalize the new behaviors you are trying to instill. Mental energy gives you the resolve to perform the actions required to facilitate the rewiring of your brain.

Pathological overeaters are fixated in a heavy, negative, habitual brain rut rooted in their ancient reptilian brain. Dr. John Ratey, in his book *Spark (The Revolutionary New Science of Exercise and the Brain),* says that this pathological behavior is caused by people instinctively trying to satiate their intense desire for pleasure from eating.[11] Mitigate this type of behavior by using your conscious intentions to infuse your subconscious toward adopting a more measured outcome.

Dr. Wayne Dyer speaks to these points in his book *Excuses Begone*. Dyer says that our habitual, subconscious brain causes us to spend a lot of time on auto-pilot and takes care of much of what we think, say or do. But our subconscious programming can be re-written. Everything you speak, say or do is ultimately a choice that you can control. When you choose to ignore your conscious beliefs, your habitual subconscious always takes over. However, you can shift your conscious brain to explore and choose your options.[12]

The Take 5 tool is a perfect way to rapidly and easily shift your response mode to your conscious brain. Take 5 is a highly effective shortcut to blunt an immediate craving impulse and ensures that you can effect permanent long-run changes.

The Power of Creating a Deliberate Intention to Change

If you infuse your subconscious with your rational, willful intentions, you change your mind-set and learn to respond to environmental stimuli, psychosocial cues and triggers in a less destructive way. This falls in the province of the last and newest part of your brain, the neocortex. It is in the neocortex that the rational and analytical parts of your brain are housed.[13] It is through the use of your conscious, rational mind that you can modify and control your emotional self.

The first part of reducing your accessibility to food and snacks involves changing your mind-set and creating the intentions you need to modify your lifestyle in a more moderate and healthy manner. To modify your behavior, you first have to create a conscious intention to change.[14] While this may seem obvious, you need to do it in a real and believable way. First, write down your intention in as exact and precise language as you can. For example:

> *"My intention is to change my lifestyle in a realistic and sustainable way that allows me to eat healthier, eat less, to better control my long-term weight level."*

With a little more effort, you can transform your intention and make it into a full-blown personal mission statement.[15] With introspection and deep thought, ask yourself why you want this intention to become a reality. Is it to find a more attractive partner or a date, to give you more energy, because you want to be alive to see your children live well into adulthood, or is it something else? Whatever it is, try to identify the real driver(s) of your intention.

Writing down your intention to change reinforces the willpower you need to make these changes in a manner that minimizes the depletion of your mental energy. If you try to keep this thought uppermost in your mind at all times, it requires great vigilance and effort, which depletes your mental energy and weakens your willpower. It is better to write it down and refer to it frequently (e.g., pre-bed and maybe upon awakening in the morning).

The Placebo Effect and the Power of Positive Expectations

One critical and often underappreciated tool that you can use to bolster your resolve is to understand the role of expectations on your behavior.[16] The placebo effect is an incredibly powerful force that creates a reality out of your beliefs of what is possible, what can be achieved and what is likely to occur. It is well-known that the placebo effect accounts for a very significant part of the healing process and the overall efficacy of medical drug therapy. In the same way and via the same brain circuits, you must expect that your intentions are doable and that you have the ability to make them happen.[17] Belief in your ability to effect change and the conscious reiteration of this belief is a tactic that reinforces your mental energy. Self-doubt saps your confidence and willpower, whereas self-validation boosts it.

You must do what you can to connect to your subconscious emotions and inform your subconscious mind that you not only want something to happen, but believe you can create this reality. The power of a placebo is often dismissed as not very important. Even while using your rational, conscious self to try and influence your subconscious, the power of positive expectations is critical. Change may occur without a definite belief that you can effect such change, but it is very unlikely to occur if you truly doubt you have the stuff to make it happen. This is one reason that Take 5 is so powerful and so effective. It is highly credible and believable as a tool to defuse an emotional impulse, and this belief actually helps it to work even better.

The Power of the Placebo Effect

Credible evidence supporting the power of the placebo effect can be found in research from the Harvard Medical School. In this study, the researchers gave migraine headache sufferers deliberately mislabeled pills. They labeled the real migraine relief drug a dummy placebo and labeled the dummy placebo pill a real drug. The surprising result was that those receiving the placebo labeled as a real drug experienced double the pain relief as reported by those who received the real drug labeled as a placebo. The patients' expectations completely overwhelmed the power of the actual drug in producing a real (albeit self-reported) effect. The placebo effect is real, and it is very strong.

So powerful is the placebo effect that Newberg and Waldman, in their book *How God Changes Your Brain,* state "even an irrational belief in a cure proven not to work can significantly boost the body's immune system when dealing with a deadly disease."[21] Since the placebo effect has this kind of power, you should utilize it to help effect the behavioral changes you want to realize in your lifestyle.

I have a real life story of my own that validates the power of the placebo effect. I started smoking when I was 15 years old. By the time I was 35, I was tired of the filth, stink and costs associated with smoking. I tried to quit at least a half dozen times, it never worked for more than a few weeks. It is now known that nicotine is one of the most addicting drugs. Fortunately, I literally stumbled onto a possible solution in a magazine. It was an advertisement promoting the use of hypnosis to help break habits, including the urge to smoke.

The use of hypnosis was then (1982) and is still now, controversial. Some scientists and psychologists dismiss its ability to permanently change our behavior and deem it a hoax. But I was a total believer. I always believed that the human mind is capable of incredible feats, including being able to exert total control over the body and the mind. The ad was for a local, hypnosis seminar and promised to break one's smoking habit in one three hour session. I immediately signed up and persuaded three other friends who smoked to join me.

The hypnosis seminar was led by a hypnotherapist and attended by a total of 15 participants. The first two hours he spoke about hypnosis and how powerful and effective it was in changing behavior (this, of course, fed right into my own pre-existing expectations about its power to effect change). The last hour involved the actual hypnotic induction. The therapist recommended that we lie down on the carpeted floor for maximum relaxation and receptivity. Only one person chose to lie down and that was me. The therapist spoke in a calm and reassuring voice about how we could easily stop smoking without any unintended consequences, like weight gain. An hour that felt like a few minutes, passed quickly and then the seminar was over.

The next day I awoke and went to work without any thought of lighting-up. That day at lunch in the company cafeteria, I saw people smoking (yes, it was still allowed back then) and thought how odd they appeared to me, still without any inclination to light-up myself. Now, more than 38 years later, I not only have not ever smoked another cigarette, I have not had the slightest urge to do so.

Interestingly, all three of my friends claimed to have been hypnotized, but only the two of us who had a strong expectation and pre-existing belief in the power of hypnosis were actually successful.

Persistence Is Key

Positive belief in your ability to effect fundamental changes in your lifestyle makes such changes much more likely to occur. Persistence is the key! As Nobel Prize winning psychologist Daniel Kahneman says in his book *Thinking Fast and Slow,* "optimism encourages persistence in the face of obstacles."[18] Your belief in a positive outcome makes it much more likely to occur by providing a natural boost in the mental energy that supports your willpower and self-control.

In order to build positive expectations, it is beneficial to repeat to yourself the following types of statements. For example:

- "Setbacks are temporary and can be overcome!"
- "I will eat sensibly today and consciously choose what I will consume."
- "I will consciously choose when and where I eat a high-sugar and/or high-simple-carb food."
- "When faced with a *Fat* Brain versus *Skinny* brain choice, (*Your Name*) will always Take 5 and choose to follow his/her *Skinny* brain."

By repeating these statements, you can increase their value and efficacy. Harvard Business School professor Amy Cuddy wrote a book called *Presence.*[19] She discusses how the use of power posing stances can change how you feel and subsequently how you behave. Repeat the previous statements while standing in a power posing position. A typical power pose is where you stand with your feet apart, your hands on your hips, and your chin tilted upward.

Cuddy provides evidence that such a pose can increase your confidence. A boost in confidence gives you a boost in your conviction that you can follow through on the desired behaviors described in the statements that you are repeating. Remember the power of positive expectations. When you have a belief in a particular outcome, it is far likelier to occur. When you believe in the value of power posing, it makes it a self-fulfilling prophecy.

It may sound somewhat like New Age psychobabble, but, there is a definite truth to the premise that you can become the person you want to be by consciously striving to live your life as you want it to become and downloading this desire to your subconscious.[20]

Your Journey to Transformational Diet Lifestyle Change

You must accept that the path to achieving significant, long-term, behavioral change is not a straight line. During the journey toward your ultimate goal, you will encounter plateaus, reversals and dead ends that may seem insurmountable. You may feel like you have failed. These are setbacks, not failures, Use them as learning experiences. Consciously think about the setback and discuss it with your partner or best friend. Review your recent behavior and try to discern what cues caused your behavior to deviate from your goal. By identifying your own idiosyncratic trigger points, you learn to better avoid them in the future.

Always keep in mind the critical overarching mantra, "Your brain is the master of your behavior and YOU are the master of your brain." The power is in your hands and brain to change. A setback, if you fall off the healthy eating bandwagon, does not have to derail the whole transformation train. It may slow your arrival to your final destination, it may re-route you along the way, but you will get there eventually.

The Role of Perceptual Reframing

One of the most critical actions you can take to control overeating, inappropriate snacking and consuming too much sugar and simple carbs, is to reframe your thinking about snacking.[22] For far too many people a meal, at least dinner (and maybe including lunch) is not complete without dessert. Dessert to most people means a sugary, high-calorie food. Research strongly supports the notion that totally eliminating any food, even high-sugar foods, from your diet is not sensible and often self-defeating.[23] To try and deny your brain's craving for sweets 100% of the time seldom works.

But here is where you can use your brain to reframe dessert, and in particular, high-calorie, high-sugar desserts from a daily consumption event to a special treat status. For example, instead of a daily high-sugar dessert, have a once-a-week special dessert occasion. I personally favor a special dessert for Sunday evening dinners. You still have something to look forward to and make that dinner occasion into a special event. If you reposition dessert to a once-weekly treat, you greatly reduce your consumption of such foods without sacrificing its enjoyment. Of course, there are also other very special celebratory events where having a sweet, sugary dessert is OK. For those very limited occasions where you have a birthday, anniversary, or any really special occasion, a dessert does not harm your health or your adherence to following the Whole Brain Diet Lifestyle.

Limiting dessert is a great sustaining tactic that maintains your mental energy. If you know with certainty that you have a sugary dessert at least once per week, it is easier to bypass the urge on a daily basis. This means you do not need to use as much mental energy to sustain your vigilance, and more mental energy is available to resist other unplanned temptations that come your way.

In making the transition to a weekly, special treat occasion, it may help to substitute some sweet fruits or low-sugar frozen treats as an alternative dessert. Or even better, replace them with whole, fresh, locally grown fruit in season.

Reframing Example from the Author's Life
When I was a new college graduate with a good-paying job and a new bride, I had certain long-held ideas about food. One of these perceptions was that as a sign of good taste and a symbol of affluence, you could not beat having a thick, juicy steak for dinner. This was the epitome of an excellent meal, and one I looked forward to frequently. Over the years as the hidden dangers of saturated fat and over-grilling became more known, my perceptions about the ideal meal evolved. I started to think of steak and beef as an occasional treat rather than a more frequent entree. Interestingly, the emotional imagery I now associate with eating steak has also changed appreciably. The thought of eating a steak no longer fires up my sensory reward circuits as it once did. I no longer crave it, and I consume it infrequently. As the pleasure and reward value of eating beef diminished, I reframed my perception of steak or beef from a twice weekly event to enjoying it once a month. I began to perceive meat to be a heavy food and realized that minimizing its consumption is one facet of following a lite approach to life.

The point is that you have the power to change long-held perceptions about what desirable food is, and, more importantly, to change your lifestyle to position some foods as being most appropriate to enjoy only occasionally.

You can use, as I did, your conscious deliberate brain to alter your subconscious emotional associations. Your brain and your perceptions are malleable and can be altered.[24] Changing your mind-set provides a powerful sustaining strategy that minimizes depletion of your mental energy and self-control by removing a frequent temptation to consume high-sugar, high-simple-carb and other high-calorie foods from your daily life.

Reframing Your Food Choices

Your predisposition favoring sweet foods and rejecting bitter ones is mostly instinctive, but most of the rest of what you prefer is learned. If these preferences are learned, then it follows that you have the power to unlearn them and form new food preferences. How do you do this?

I've found interesting and novel way to tolerate and even look forward to new food experiences. It's a way that promotes heightened acceptance and greater consumption of certain foods. This employs an anti-confirmation bias. Many of you have likely heard of the term confirmation bias. It is the human tendency to seek out and accept ideas, information and data which confirms your pre-existing beliefs and to reject much of what does not do this. Anti-confirmation bias turns this idea upside down.

For example, you may want to eat more healthful foods and believe that eating a lot more vegetables helps you to achieve this goal. Use your willful intent to actively, daily, seek out news stories and research that proves or reinforces the idea that veggies are very healthful and that their consumption offers many benefits to the body and mind. Also, seek to find delicious new ways to serve them (e.g., I recently discovered low-sugar, very low-calorie, fresh yogurt-based dressings that are delicious and perfect for dipping raw veggies). This behavior, over time, strengthens your perceptions of the value and advantages of eating vegetables and these perceptions actually propel you to try new vegetables and new vegetable recipes.

Our expectations have a powerful influence on how we actually perceive an experience, including eating foods that are new to us or that we seldom typically consume. Knowing and believing that vegetables are super-healthy and having an expectation that their taste is tolerable, if not enjoyable, can change your feelings about eating them and this causes you to eat them more often.

You can use your conscious intent to repeatedly seek and consume pro-vegetable information in a way that actually changes your perceptions. Your perceptions help to build your attitudes and beliefs and these shape your behavior. You have the power to change your food preferences and hence your food choices.

For myself, I once held very negative perceptions about yogurt. I thought that it was an uninteresting food, with a boring unsatisfying taste and mouth feel. What's more, I wrongfully thought of it as a food more for women, than men. Over time I heard pro-health comments about yogurt, like the probiotics they contain, and decided to actively seek to learn more about it. I looked for news and research about how healthy yogurt is. Then, by adding other healthful foods to the yogurt, like a small amount of walnuts or whole grain cereal, I changed my perceptions and subsequently my attitudes, so that I began to eat it more and enjoy it more. Today, I eat no fat, no sugar added yogurt almost every day. As the pundits say, "mind over matter".

Forming Habits

In his book *The Power of Habit,* Charles Duhigg says that our habits are powered by a process of psychosocial and physical cues, prompting a habitual response that generates a reward for the brain, reinforcing the habitual response. But he identifies a facilitating factor needed to make this process work: a craving. Following the initial cue that triggers the response, but before the habitual response, there must be a craving that anticipates the brain reward to follow and the expected satisfaction to be realized.[25]

In the instant between cue and response, the brain's anticipation of reward actually causes us to behave in a manner that over time becomes ingrained and automatic. How does all of this relate to how you change and reframe your perceptions?

If the sight and sound of a sizzling steak in a television commercial does not fire off a fleeting anticipatory reward signal associated with consuming this food, then a craving is not likely to be generated, and you are unlikely to follow through by eating a steak.

When I see a commercial for a steak restaurant, or a high-simple-carb/high-sugar food, my immediate brain reaction is subdued, even negative, as my initial perception is that the unhealthful nature of these items overwhelms the taste and sensory pleasure I would get from eating them. The intense, old craving is not there, or is much diminished, so the old habitual response is much less likely to be activated. The key is what happens in the moment, in the very instant when the stimulus presents itself. Change the initial reaction to the moment, and you change the subsequent behavior.

Mental repetition, reinforced by exposure to negative messages or images related to unhealthful foods or snacks (like steak or high-simple-carb, high-sugar foods), can alter your brain circuits. By altering your subconscious associations, the intrinsic appeal of such foods is naturally diminished, and the ability of the old food cues to trigger the same old automatic consumption response is broken.

Habits Can Be Highly Productive

For many, your perceptions regarding the word habit is that its connotation is primarily negative. We all have some habits that we wish to break and are better off without. But habits are not necessarily negative. Habits are modes of decision-making and/or behavior that have become routine and essentially automatic in response to a particular stimuli. Habits can be an incredibly powerful and efficient way to behave. If we consciously strive to make it so, a habit can be a huge positive, with real benefits to your brain and to your life. We often fret so much about our bad habits that we forget to try to build really good, productive ones.

Habitual behaviors make us feel comfortable and often ease tension (at least initially). To break a habit and create new ones, you must learn to tolerate and accept a temporary state of discomfort. The longer you have had the habitual behavior and the more important a role it plays in your life, the more entrenched it is, and the greater the discomfort you feel when trying to break it. How can you get through this transition period? You need some ways to lessen the discomfort you typically feel. Practicing mindfulness is an excellent tool that you can nurture with the following activities:

- When you feel discomfort, be mindful enough to recognize it. Label it as a discomfort you feel because you are working to replace an old habit. The very act of labeling reduces the intensity of an emotional experience and allows it to lose its momentum and dissipate more quickly.
- Take actions to increase your normal stress management practices. For example, amp up your exercise routine, listen to more music, read a book or meditate.
- Do not just sit there and experience the tension and discomfort without any intervention. Work off your nervous energy to distract yourself and to focus on the benefits of the new habit.

Use Take 5 to reduce the discomfort you feel while you are trying to deny a craving, by taking a proactive step that reduces the stress that comes with feeling discomfort. After employing Take 5 for a few months using Take 5 becomes habitual and the discomfort you feel from trying to break your snacking habit is greatly diminished.

Willpower, Resolve and Resisting Temptation

Before you have reframed your thinking and changed your mind-set, you probably feel that resisting a high-sugar, high-calorie snack is simply a matter of exercising your willpower. You may blame giving in to an impulse to indulge on not having enough willpower and resolve. Recent research into the science of willpower shows your willpower is highest in the morning and at its maximum level early in the day.[26] As you tire and as you expend mental and physical energy on work or other endeavors, your willpower diminishes.[27]

It takes a great deal of awareness to constantly defer or deny an urge that resides in your subconscious.[28] The longer you try to remain vigilant against a snack-attack, the more difficult it becomes to dispel the urge as your willpower wanes.[29]

Envisioning Your Future Self: An Important Cognitive Bias

Another important way in which you can increase your willpower and resolve is to increase your recognition and awareness of your likely or possible future self. Kelly McGonigal in her book *The Willpower Instinct* says that people need to try to better understand and appreciate how their future health and well-being depends on the decisions and behaviors they choose today and every day.[30] As I like to say, "Today is yesterday's tomorrow." The actions and decisions you make at each point in time creates the life you face and enjoy in the future.

One very important reason that willpower alone is not enough is that many people are unable to adequately link their potential future health to their present-day behaviors due to a cognitive bias. Cognitive biases are mind-sets and ingrained ways of thinking that are distorted by some belief or mental framework that is not true. You probably have a strong predisposition to discount the likelihood of future risks that are remote, vague or simply far removed from your present circumstance as though they will never occur.

This cognitive bias allows you to continue to behave in ways that may harm you in the distant future, like unhealthful overeating, smoking or not exercising. The present-day consequences of these actions seem limited and not highly concerning. The risks associated with these behaviors, which are known to your conscious mind as precursors to potential future obesity, diabetes, cancer or heart disease, are severely underestimated.

This particular cognitive bias is firmly grounded in our evolutionary history. On the plains of pre-historic Africa or during the era of the caveman, survival was day to day. Immediate existential threats from predators, other humans or starvation were ever-present. Man had to focus on his immediate environment to maximize his chances of surviving. Paying attention to the vague and unknown risks of a remote future was not, at that time, brain-smart or life-preserving. In those days and over much of our evolutionary history, maintaining a very short-term focus was the right thing to do and most consistent with self-preservation behavior.

This cognitive bias has real consequences. One of them is that we delude ourselves into thinking that the distant future will never arrive and that we do not have to deal with the future consequences of our immediate behaviors. Interestingly, there is a somewhat quirky method that you can use to help defuse this bias and make you much more aware of the future and how your actions in the present can affect your future health and well-being. Oddly enough, it is to consciously think about and even record your thoughts and feelings about death and dying.

This act has the ability to focus your attention on an inevitability that we all face sometime and how our present behaviors may prematurely hasten this eventuality. The point is to nudge your behavior in the direction of making decisions and taking actions that are consistent with your longer-term goals and to help promote your conscious goal of achieving real dietary lifestyle transformation. Serendipitously, this action puts your life into a different and more useful perspective and changes your attitudes and behaviors in other complementary areas as well.

Connecting Future Scenarios to Your Present Self

What implications does this have for how you can motivate yourself to follow the Whole Brain Diet Lifestyle in today's world? You need a mechanism to better connect your behaviors in the present to future risk scenarios. Focus not only on the dire potential future health consequences of your present-day behaviors, but also on the current emotional and psychosocial consequences of these behaviors on your present reality and your future life.

What does this mean? Let's take the example of overeating, which may cause you to gain weight and become obese. Instead of trying to relate only to the future health risks associated with obesity, governmental public service campaigns and the medical profession should also emphasize the negative social impact of obesity on one's likelihood of finding an ideal partner and mate. Most of us have an innate drive to find a life partner to facilitate the replication of our DNA via our offspring or just to satisfy our evolutionary-based need for intimacy and a deep personal connection to another being. Harness this instinct to better highlight the more immediate risks of overeating on your life and on your future happiness. This boosts your willpower and self-control by relating the consequences to your present life, not some distant, vague and unknowable future.

Instead of reaching for that extra piece of bread, that second helping of spaghetti or that larger piece of cake, visualize your body getting larger and fatter and the impact on your future social life and desirability as a mate for a potential suitor or as a lover for your partner. If you already have a life partner, think about the impact of getting fatter on the likelihood that you can sustain and keep that partnership alive and vital in the long-run. Non-health risks may be more compelling and more motivating than focusing only on future, potential negative health consequences. Obviously, your waist doesn't actually get bigger with every bite of food you consume. You can, however, use the power of your imagination and your ability to visualize and to feel this sensation.

Before you eat an inappropriate, unhealthful food or snack, literally look down at your belly and visualize it getting bigger. Do you really want or need that food or snack you are contemplating? Also, keep a picture of yourself at either a healthy weight level or just a healthier level, no matter how long ago it was taken. Pull it out to remind yourself of the future shape you are striving for and of the overall lite approach to life you are trying to follow.

Constructing Your Personal Environment

When you get home at night and on the weekends, do not immediately change into your loose, expansive casual clothes that not only hide your waistline from your view, but allow you to feel completely comfortable with your waist so that you feel like you can easily consume a second helping of dinner, or a dessert or a post-dinner snack without feeling it.

You need to create your own personal environment to nudge you to behave in a manner that is consistent with your longer-term behavioral goals. Make these negative behaviors (e.g., overeating or inappropriate snacking) more deliberate and less automatic, by making your body more sensitive and responsive. There is more on the impact of sensory effects on your thoughts and behavior in Chapter 17 on "embodied cognition."

The Fat Bottle

You can even play tricks on your brain to get it to drive your behavior away from a negative choice and toward a more positive outcome. One of these useful tricks is the Fat Bottle.

The Fat Bottle is a large, transparent glass bottle, capped with an airtight lid that is filled with simulated or real fat. I recommend that you get one and place it in in your direct line-of-sight in the kitchen and by your television. It can provide a powerful cue, a visual mantra, to dissuade you from consuming an unhealthful snack, a second unnecessary portion at dinner or endless mindless snacking while watching TV. This visual cue is somewhat repulsive, but it can provide a constant reminder that the junk foods you are considering eating are readily converted to fat in your body. It also provides a powerful reminder of the fat you are trying to lose or the fat person you do not want to become.

The rationale behind the Fat Bottle is relatively simple. You encounter a stimulus like mealtime or a potential high-calorie snacking occasion; you are exposed to the visual Fat Bottle cue and the psychological response elicited is one of avoidance or moderation. The goal is not to eliminate all unhealthful eating choices, it is to make such eating less automatic and less mindless.

Further, after you feel comfortable that you have achieved real, long-run dietary transformation in your life, have a little ritualistic ceremony with your close friends and family to bury the Fat Bottle (or otherwise discard it). This provides a further reassurance that your quest for behavioral transformation succeeded, and this aid is no longer required.

Why Visual Mantras Work

Visual mantras work because they simply, yet powerfully, encapsulate and communicate a message that you recall when given an appropriate cue. In this case, the cue may be any meal or snack occasion in which you might be tempted by unhealthful foods. What is the perfect mantra? It is one that is always accessible, always visible at the moment of maximum vulnerability when you must make a decision to give in or avoid a temptation. In this vein, there is another powerful visual mantra that is highly useful to reinforce your willpower in the moment when you need it the most.

This new visual mantra uses the popularity and ever-present visibility of a wrist band to communicate the intended message. Specifically, buy a rubberized wristband in a soft, calming color (like light blue) inscribed with the bolded message: **EAT SMART – EAT IN MODERATION.** Wear this wristband whenever you are awake, so it is present during all occasions where food consumption is possible. You could also wear a second wristband emblazoned with a bold imprint that says simply, **TAKE 5.** Links to where you can order these are available on our website www.take5diet.com.

Why do these visual mantras work? In essence, by continually wearing the wristbands, you can employ the power of operant conditioning to train your brain. Say you experience a cue, like a craving to eat a high-sugar, high-calorie snack. This stimuli elicits a response to look at your wristband. You should not only look down at your wristband you should tap it as this act, metaphorically speaking, activates and energizes your Take 5 response and initiates the Take 5 process. You can then consciously decide to side with your *Skinny* brain long enough for the initial craving to subside or completely dissipate. Over time, the mere presence of the wristband itself is enough to activate the Take 5 response without your actually being aware of the band itself. Using operant conditioning, you train your brain to respond naturally and automatically to provide enough time for your snack-attack craving to go away.

How does it work? The band works like a meme that can infect your brain with a healthy message that becomes internalized over time. Think of it as the modern-day equivalent of tying a string around your finger as a reminder to do something, only this string has a very specific message emblazoned on it. The more you wear it, the more you see it, the more potential effect it has. What's more, it can also act to motivate your friends and acquaintances who may also absorb the message and become natural reinforcing agents in helping to make it work for you. This visual mantra is easy, it's simple, it's inexpensive, and it can be highly effective.

Role of Simplifying Your Life

Your brain loves constancy and routine, and as such it abhors complexity that makes decision making more difficult and riskier. You can simplify your life by reducing uncertainty, the number of decisions that you need to make and the number of options you have to choose from. Certainty and simplicity make your brain happy.

How can you simplify your life? One key strategy is to pre-schedule and pre-plan your life along as many dimensions as possible. When you do this, you do not need to expend as much mental energy deciding what to do next or how to proceed at any point in time. Routine builds the neuronal network in your brain, making the interconnections stronger and more robust.

Plan your week and especially your day with a clear schedule of activities. This includes always creating a daily planning list every night before bedtime so you have an idea, at least on paper, of how your day will unfold. This simplifies your life each day and reduces unnecessary time and anxiety on how to proceed.

You might go so far as to plan your break times, snack times, mealtimes, and downtime. This creates an aura of certainty, even if events preclude your following the plan. This helps you prevent unnecessary depletion of your mental energy and hence better maintain your willpower, resolve and self-control.

Pre-scheduling your meal and snack times gives your brain a reassurance that food and nourishment is coming. The instinct to eat resides in your ancient reptilian brain and commands your attention and priority over those generated by the higher-order conscious part of your brain. When you are hungry, or just thinking about food, your attention is diffused, your willpower is diminished, and your likelihood of giving in to a snack-attack is magnified. Additionally, if you are at work, your productivity and creativity is reduced as some of your focus is diverted to your stomach. Pre-scheduling also reduces your likelihood of becoming hangry!

Along this same line of reasoning, a specific meal plan can be highly beneficial. This is especially true for breakfast, when time is short. I eat the same basic breakfast every day (flavors and varieties change, but the components of the meal remain the same). I always keep the ingredients available and never have to waste time trying to decide what to eat. As a consequence, my day always gets started with a complete, nutritious breakfast.

The Genius of Facebook's Mark Zuckerberg

It's not only breakfast where following the same routine is a brain-smart and beneficial behavior. Mark Zuckerberg is the founder/CEO of the immensely successful company Facebook. One behavior he has adopted is to wear the same outfit every workday. He does this, he says, because it is easy and requires no hard, unnecessary thinking early in the morning. Zuckerberg's behavior is very brain-smart and conserves mental energy. The challenges of daily living deplete your mental energy throughout a normal day, and whatever you can do to conserve it makes it more likely to be available when you really need it – like to avoid a tempting, ultra-processed snack at your mid-morning or afternoon break. You should consider doing so because it simply makes sense and helps to sustain your mental energy.

The Fallacy of Multi-tasking

Another facet of simplifying your life is learning to focus totally on one activity at a time. Many of us pride ourselves on our ability to multi-task. However, brain science indicates that we are kidding ourselves to think that we can really do this effectively.[31] Trying to focus on multiple tasks at one time adds complexity to our lives, and this complexity stresses the brain in a way that increases the depletion of your mental energy. Multi-tasking usually provides for less effective outcomes. Focusing on one task at a time is also a very useful sustaining tactic. It simplifies your life, reduces stress, and lessens the depletion of your mental energy.

The Panic-Button Tool (aka the emotional circuit breaker)

You can create and reinforce your intention to change, including changing your mind-set to reframe the dessert occasion. You can try to use your willpower to resist a snack, but sometimes you will not succeed. At some point you will be sorely tempted to succumb to your cravings. How can you counter this inevitable urge to cheat? One tactic is to employ the panic-button technique as an emotional circuit breaker to defuse, or at least delay, giving in to a snack-attack urge.

To paraphrase the Buddha, the secret of health for both mind and body is not to mourn for the past, not to worry about the future, or not to anticipate troubles, but to live the present moment wisely and earnestly. You can change a habitual response or behavior only in the moment when you feel the urge to act on your habit.[32] Defusing an urge or craving to eat is no different. If you can detach yourself and observe your emotional impulse, it loses its momentum.[33] This is why the panic-button technique dramatically affects your behavior and ability to be mindful of what you eat.

There are up to six steps you may follow to use this tool. For most of you, employing Step 1 alone is likely enough.

Step 1 is to invoke and use the Take 5 technique. Exhale fully, then take five deep, deep breaths and exhale slowly while silently repeating the Take 5 mantra. All you may need is a moment to interrupt the emotional urge to consume right now. This allows you to consciously decide to go lite and to follow the dictates of your *Skinny* brain. This simple practice may allow the urge to snack unhealthfully or to overeat to dissipate as many cravings are very fleeting.[34]

If this immediate time delay circuit-breaker is not effective, you can proceed to Step 2. In this phase, you resort to pulling out and reading a card with statements on it, such as:

- "(*Your Name*) does not give in to this craving for a high-calorie, high-sugar snack."
- "(*Your Name*) chooses not to eat an unhealthy snack at this time."
- "(*Your Name*)'s time to eat high-sugar, high-calorie snacks are for weekend desserts only."
- "(*Your Name*) continues to follow a lite lifestyle that limits inappropriate, unhealthful snacking."

This may serve as a quick, emergency aid to bolster your willpower and resolve allowing you to resist a momentary temptation.

Step 3 is to try to break your snack-attack impulse using a quick (e.g., 5 to 10 minutes) of standing up and moving around.[35] Exercise, or any physical activity, offers the following benefits to help reduce or eliminate an urge to snack:

- A distraction that diverts your attention away from your craving.
- An alternative means of rewarding your brain with physical activity rather than an unhealthful snack.
- A break from routine to recognize that a negative emotion such as anger, boredom or loneliness may have precipitated your snack-attack and that you are not truly hungry.

Step 4 is to use your brain to trick your brain. Try a thought or visualization exercise in which you actively imagine that you are eating the unhealthful snack that you are trying to avoid. This imaginary exercise can trigger a real response in your brain by lighting up your brain's reward circuits similarly to actually indulging in eating a real food. Research indicates that imagining and/or remembering an activity invokes a similar emotion and brain-state as really engaging in the physical activity and release brain chemicals like dopamine that make you feel good.[36]

In Step 5, you can fall back on the social power of calling a spouse or friend for moral support (of course you would set this up ahead of time).[37] This may allow them to talk you down from the proverbial ledge to safer ground where you no longer want to eat a snack.

Step 6, if you still desire a snack of some type, you can reach for a healthful alternative, like a piece of fruit or vegetable and yogurt dip. You should always keep these types of foods readily accessible.

The whole purpose of the panic-button tool is to break the emotional momentum that is propelling you to snack inappropriately and unhealthfully during an unplanned, non-deliberate occasion. This tool may not always work, but it makes your reaching for and consuming an unhealthful snack less automatic, more deliberate, and more mindful. If you still choose to have a high-calorie snack, at least it is a more conscious choice, not simply a knee-jerk reaction to an emotional cue or trigger.

The panic-button technique is effective because it gives a critical boost to your mental energy and hence your self-control just at the moment of maximum vulnerability when you need it the most.

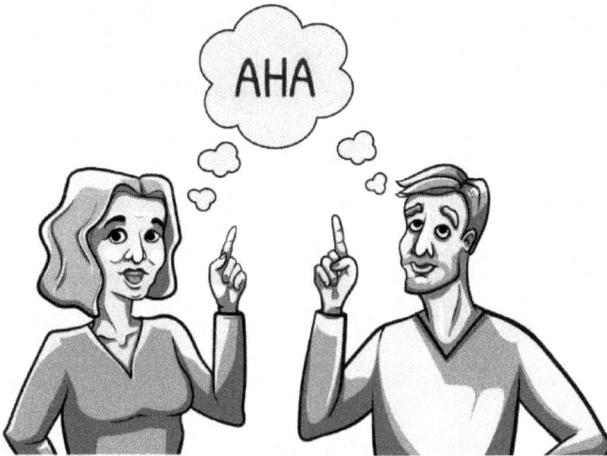

- In the exact moment you experience a craving, you always have a choice to yield to it or not. Every craving provides an opportunity to squash it, however briefly. If you nurture your ability to be self-aware and mindful, you can give yourself an extra second to consciously react to the craving, before you respond in a more reflexive, automatic manner. One of the best ways to generate the mindful awareness you need to make a deliberate choice is by using the Take 5 technique.

- Substituting a positive, healthy habit for an unhealthy, negative one is not rocket science, but it does take persistence and perseverance that is powered by your mental energy and a belief that you have the ability to make the change happen. Your expectations, either positive or negative, have a powerful impact on your behavior. Optimism helps to power you through the obstacles you meet on your journey to achieving a transformational change to your diet lifestyle.

Chapter 10: Social Barriers
Your brain craves and needs affiliation, friendship and sharing, like roses need rain, in order to bloom and flourish.

There are several important pieces to the puzzle of making food and snacking less accessible by using social influences.

Impact of a Public Pledge on Realizing Change
In addition to intending to change your lifestyle, make it known to your spouse, significant others, relatives, and friends.[1] Tell them you intend to change your relationship to food and your overall food consumption behavior. This can be done informally. But it is also a good idea to put your intention into writing or emailing your friends and / or posting your intentions to social media. In this way, these other people help you transform your intent into a reality.

Another important pledge you can make to yourself is to pledge to make using the Take 5 technique your first response to an emotional impulse to eat unhealthfully. Reinforce using Take 5 every day by telling yourself, "(*Your Name*) pledges to always Take 5 before he/she responds to a snack craving."

Research shows that making a pledge, both private and public, affects your making it real and achievable.[2] When you make a pledge, you increase the importance of trying to follow through on your intention to change, as you do not want to disappoint others and are often eager to receive their praise and good wishes.

Enlisting the Cooperation of Others
Equally important, your pledge alerts your significant others to help you avoid temptation and to avoid putting you in situations where it is difficult not to overeat or eat unhealthfully. Creating a pledge increases the likelihood of your succeeding in carrying out the changes in your lifestyle that you want to realize. If you ask others for their help, you effectively make achieving a lifestyle transformation a shared goal and thereby more achievable.

The pledge assures that your spouse/partner/friends/colleagues are aware of your intent to change; are more likely to support your intention; and helps you to structure an environment in which such change is more readily accommodated and temptations to resist change are avoided or minimized. Enlisting the support of others allows you to use their willpower, instead of only your own, to keep you on the path toward the behavioral change(s) you want to achieve.

Of course, even better than a pledge to assure the aid and support of a partner/friend/colleague, is to ask someone to join you in your challenge to adopt a healthier Whole Brain Diet Lifestyle. There is no better way to do this than having a significant other accompany you on your quest.

When you engage others, who are important to you to join you, then you also automatically activate the power of social persuasion in realizing your behavioral change goals. When you and your partner/friend(s) share the same end game, the likelihood of successfully achieving your goal increases significantly.[3] You can multiply your willpower by a factor of two (or more).

No one wants to let down a partner or friend, and no one can provide more natural and heartfelt encouragement to continue striving than they can. Your desire to avert a failure is much more powerful in the presence and awareness of those whose opinions you care about.

Social connectivity and approval are craved by the brain, so enlisting social relationships to further your goal of achieving behavioral change is very brain-smart. When you engage your significant others in your mission, a happy brain releases neurotransmitters such as dopamine and oxytocin, which reward you with positive, uplifting feelings. This reward to your brain provides additional incentive to continue on your path and persevere long enough to establish new habitual, behavioral responses aligned with your conscious goals.

You should also try to avoid or minimize interaction and socialization with negative people. Choose to spend more time with positive people, who are lite in spirit, in mood and in weight. Obesity is said to be contagious, and so is thinness. Associate more with lite people, and it will be easier for you to be lite yourself, including following a lite diet lifestyle.

Impact of Psychosocial and Emotional Cues
When you are trying to change your lifestyle and achieve a weight loss, it is beneficial to avoid or at least minimize coming into contact with

psychosocial and other cues that may automatically encourage unhealthy snacking or overeating.[4]

Such cues may include physical situations, such as:

- Going to parties
- Eating a meal in a restaurant
- Sitting down and watching television
- Going to a movie theater
- Going to a sporting event
- Other situations where drinking alcohol to excess may occur
- Spending time with heavy people (heavy in mood, spirit and/or weight)

All of these occasions may prompt you to eat more automatically and with less conscious thinking. While you may choose to still engage in these behaviors, if you have enough self-awareness to know that they are dangerous flash points that may prompt unhealthy eating or snacking, it is more likely that you can substantially resist the urge to eat inappropriately and/or to overeat or over-drink.

There are also emotional triggers that can prompt unhealthy and inappropriate eating, snacking, and overeating. These include situations where negative emotions are felt that may be confused or mistaken for real feelings of hunger. For example, when you experience certain emotions, you may reach for food, when your hunger is really for emotional resolution.[5]

These negative emotions include:

- Anger
- Frustration
- Loneliness
- Nervousness or tenseness
- Anxiety
- Boredom
- Guilt

Take 5 is particularly effective to counter a snack impulse that is simply a reaction to a negative emotional stimuli, not true hunger. Being self-aware and having the ability to step back, be mindful and distance yourself from an emotion allows you to discern that what you feel is an emotional urge that you need to address in other ways. Take 5 provides you with exactly the detachment, and the mental and physical distance from your emotional impulse, to do just this.

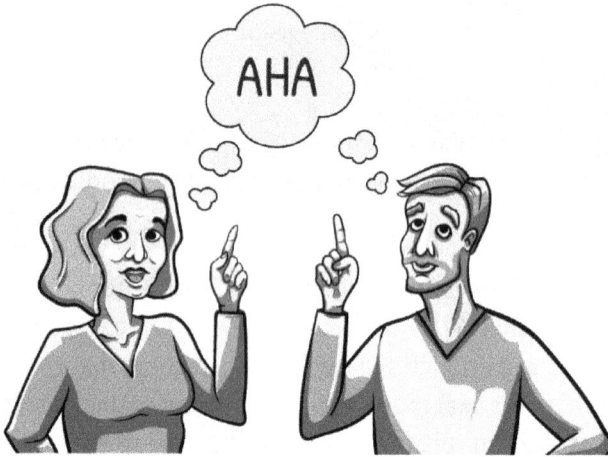

- Share your quest for dietary lifestyle transformation with a partner or friend to multiply the probability of ultimately achieving your goal. Friends and family encourage you to continue your quest, and we all seek the approval and praise they offer. Employing the power of social connectivity is evolutionarily-favored as a life preserving activity both in pre-historic times and in today's world.
- Being self-aware and mindful is a highly important attribute to nurture and grow in order to facilitate your dietary lifestyle transformation. While you might become "obsessed" with being self-aware, it is not a bad thing, and it is extremely difficult to become too self-aware.

Chapter 11: Physical Barriers

Your behavior is <u>not</u> pre-determined; you can construct your physical environment to nudge your behavior in the direction you want it to go.

This chapter is about using the most important and powerful sustaining tactics: adopting physical barriers to limit accessibility to unhealthful foods. These barriers greatly help to sustain your mental energy, your willpower and self-control, by creating a physical environment that naturally discourages consumption of these foods.

When you construct these physical barriers to reduce accessibility to high-simple-carb, high-sugar foods, you automatically reduce the number of unhealthy food decisions that you need to make. You also reduce the number of times you need to rely on the power of repeating the Take 5 mantra, reserving it for those occasions where you really need an immediate boost to your self-control. Using the mantra is highly effective, but not as effective as limiting your accessibility to unhealthy foods and avoiding temptations all together.

Let's start with a hypothetical day in your life from a food purchase and consumption perspective. At each decision point, suggestions, tips and rules to promote a healthier lifestyle are offered. Any single piece of advice has value. However, you do not need to adopt all of the advice offered to reap the benefits. The plan empowers you to select those features that work best for you. The more of this advice that you integrate into your life, the more likely you are to profoundly transform your relationship to food, your overall dietary lifestyle and consequently your life.[1]

A Hypothetical Day in Your Life
Grocery Shopping
First, pick a day and time of the week to do your primary weekly grocery shopping when you can be most mindful about what you buy. This is usually a time when your natural willpower is at its peak–in the morning and typically on a weekend.[2] This is a point when time pressure and other demands are often lessened. It is best to shop after breakfast when your belly is full and your body is satiated, when you are less distracted by the many temptations in the grocery store.[3] Interestingly, this is one time where heaviness of body is beneficial, as a full belly makes the brain less likely to be tempted.

Always start your grocery store visit with a pre-planned shopping list.[4] This list allows you to put in writing the needs dictated by your rational, deliberate, conscious brain. In this way, you can start your grocery visit with a good, solid intention of buying purposefully, with a mind toward selecting only what you really need. A list also simplifies your grocery store decision making and reduces uncertainty in the store. In the era of coronavirus reducing the time required to shop, also reduces your potential exposure. Pre-planning with a list makes it easy to focus on lite foods and to make a conscious attempt to exclude heavy foods before you are inside the modern temple of temptation. This action is a useful sustaining tactic that minimizes depletion of your mental energy and maintains your self-control.

When possible, shop with a significant other who also believes in adopting a healthy lifestyle. This person can act as a natural regulator of your impulses to stray from your list and succumb to the grocery store's many alluring temptations. All of us are a little bit more aware and willing to be rational when others we care about are with us.

In the store, plan your path around the aisles very carefully. Do not go down any aisles that are filled only with foods or snacks you have not planned to purchase.[5] This may include the snack aisle, the sugary drink beverage aisle, the ice cream and frozen treat aisle and others. When you are not tempted, you do not need to maintain a vigilance that is energy depleting, leaving you with more self-control to sustain the new behaviors you are trying to adopt.

If you do pass by some high-sugar, high-simple-carb foods, Take 5. Before you put that food in your cart, continue your shopping. After a five-minute pause, see if you still want to purchase it. There is a good chance you may decide to forgo that item.

In each shopping aisle, pay attention to the nutrition labels. These labels hold valuable nutrition information, including facts about sugar, salt, fat and calories per serving. Before you pick up a specific item or a particular brand, think about the wisdom of the popular nutrition TV host who says, "Pick this, not that."[6] You may find that an alternative item or brand satisfies your needs just as well and may offer a more nutritious solution with less sugar, salt, fat and/or calories.

Before you check out, use another Take 5 timeout, and scan the contents of your shopping cart. Use your rational, conscious brain to take a last look at what you are buying. Do you really need any of the junk food in your cart? If you decide you do not need an item, simply remove it. You can choose to use your conscious willpower and resolve to override any emotional impulses that prompted you to pick up an unnecessary and unwise item.[7] You may not thwart all of your urges, but by following the Take 5 protocol you will make fewer impulsive food purchases.

After You Get Home

Most of us give very little, if any, thought to how we unpack the food items that we purchase and where we put them, but it can make a real difference. Where you put various food items, especially the high-calorie stuff, can make these items either more, or less, readily accessible. If you make these foods less accessible, you are less likely to consume them at an unplanned or inappropriate time.[8]

Put the high-calorie snack items far away from your line of vision: in a drawer or cabinet away, if possible, from where you normally sit or stand in the kitchen. Better yet, do not store them in the kitchen. You could consider buying a separate storage cabinet or refrigerator that you keep in a space outside of the kitchen to limit easy accessibility. A space like this requires a deliberate decision to visit and access.[9]

If this is not a viable option, place these items in a very high cabinet or space that you cannot readily reach to make you think twice before grabbing for a snack. Additionally, fasten the opening with a simple lock or at least a tie string that must be physically removed.[10]

Another interesting tactic is to affix a negative image to the front and inside of the cabinet or drawer that contains your most unhealthful foods. I recommend an image that presents two eyeballs, a large pointed index finger and the capitalized word Take 5.[11] This image is a physical reminder and a psychological reinforcement as well. Just as a stop sign and the color red is automatically perceived as a symbol to stop, look and think before proceeding, this image suggests pausing and waiting before opening the drawer or cabinet and removing an unhealthful food. It presents one more barrier to easy and quick accessibility to unhealthy foods and provides a brief buffer period during which an initial urge or craving can dissipate.

It may seem simplistic, but the power of an image to affect your behavior should not be underestimated. In addition to adhering a sticky with the phrase, Take 5 and a big pointed finger to your snack drawer, I also recommend incorporating one with a big face that makes a yucky-looking, unappetizing frown. The object is to provide, however briefly, some mental distance that allows you to consciously override your craving and to choose something healthier or to choose to not eat at all. These an other images are available to print for free on our website www.take5diet.com.

I also recommend that you foil wrap all of your sugary, high-simple-carb snacks to limit their visual appeal and label them with a factual descriptor as follows. Based on their calorie content, show how many minutes of exercise it takes to burn off the number of calories that snack contains. For example, if the snack contained about 300 calories, label it, "Equals at least one hour of brisk walking." Use this as a reminder that unnecessary snacking has consequences. Observe a rough chart of calories expended for various activities for a person who weighs 180 pounds.

	Walking	Slow Freestyle Swimming	Jogging	Leisure Bicycling
15 minutes	75	150	200	80
30 minutes	150	300	400	160
1 hour	300	600	800	320
2 hours	600	1200	1600	640

Another interesting technique is to color-code the shelves of your refrigerator or cupboard using colored mats or tape.[12] For example:

- Green mats or tape on shelves holding the healthiest, lower fat, lower sugar and lower calorie foods.
- Yellow mats or tape for the foods you want to consume moderately or with caution.
- Red mats or tape for the highest-carb, highest-sugar and highest-calorie foods that you want to consume very sparingly.

Before you place these high-calorie items away, there is one more precautionary step that allows you to mitigate some of the damage if and when you decide to eat some of these foods.

Where possible, you should repackage and resize these items into much smaller individual serving units.[13] Some small packages, while presented as a single unit, could actually be multiple servings. Cut the snack item into halves or thirds, as the typical full-size serving is much larger than you need to satisfy your sweet tooth and your immediate snack-attack craving. Next, put each individually sized portion into a separate plastic bag.

Offer the other half to your partner, neighbor or friend. Or, when appropriate, simply freeze the other portion. These steps help you physically constrain yourself to ultimately consume fewer calories when you do choose to eat these types of foods.

Along with making junk foods less accessible, it is a very good idea to make healthier, low-sugar, low-calorie and high-fiber foods highly accessible at all times. You want to at least have to make a mindful and purposeful decision to consume junk food, rather than respond to a quick, and perhaps fleeting, emotional urge.[14]

Pre-Meal Routine

It is easier to break a habit in the moment before the habitual behavior is initiated. The most effective way to change a habitual response like overeating or inappropriate snacking is before the stimuli (i.e., a meal or snacking occasion) presents itself.

Prior to most meals, especially before lunch and dinner, engage in a pre-emptive self-intervention to encourage food consumption moderation and restraint. This intervention takes approximately 90 seconds to execute. The only collateral material required is a wallet-sized card (or an image on your smartphone) inscribed with several key mantras to reinforce your good intentions to eat sensibly and reasonably during your next meal.

The intervention works as follows:

- Take 60 seconds to clear the mind and relax the body by exhaling completely, then inhaling and exhaling deeply five times.
- Review and read silently (or out loud) statements such as:
  - "(Your Name) will eat smart – eat in moderation."

- o *"(Your Name)* will eat slowly and mindfully to savor every bite."
- o *"(Your Name)* will stop eating when he/she feels satisfied but not full."
- o *"(Your Name)* will Take 5 before he/she gets a second serving of food and before he/she decides whether or not to have dessert."

Other phrases you might consider using include the following types of messages. The exact ones you choose should reflect your own personal preferences based on what you find to be most persuasive. I favor the messages below:

- *"(Your Name)* rejects his/her *Fat* brain and chooses to follow his/her *Skinny* brain."
- *"(Your Name)* will eat lite, not heavy."
- *"(Your Name)* will eat slowly, mindfully and with the purpose of nourishing his/her body, not his/her emotional self."
- *"(Your Name)* is in control of his/her eating behavior; it does not control him/her."

Such psychological reinforcement boosts your self-awareness, prompting you to eat mindfully and with purpose. At the same time, it enhances your willpower and resolve to eat sensibly and moderately. It is especially valuable right before an eating occasion that typically leads to overindulgence and/or consumption of particularly unhealthful foods. These occasions include going out to a restaurant, watching a sporting event or going to a party. When you are particularly vulnerable, this type of positive reinforcement can be very useful.

Another useful, pre-meal routine is to use the power of scent and aroma as a physical stimuli to change your behavior, i.e., reduce how much you consume at mealtime. It works as follows. Immediately before you start to eat inhale deeply some sweet scents you find enjoyable, like vanilla, peppermint or strawberry. This act prompts a neurological brain response activating neurons as if you were eating real food. This phenomena, along with the food you are about to eat, speeds-up your feeling satiated and when you feel satiated, you often stop eating. Scent is an effective stimuli that invokes old memories and lights-up your brain's reward circuits. It affects your brain directly, and it is not mediated by other sensory receptors before it reaches the brain, which makes it so powerful. If you know how to employ it, scent can be a highly useful behavior influencing device.

Mealtime

Scientific research strongly reinforces the notion that breakfast, as your mother always told you, is really the most important meal of the day.[15] It sets the parameters for what and how much you eat for the rest of your day. It literally means to break-the-fast. Unless you have snacked overnight, then you have not eaten any food for ten or more hours. Your body's blood sugar is running low. Your body needs to refuel. This requires you to consume calories.

Research also indicates that skipping breakfast may be dangerous to your health and even to your life. Harvard School of public health scientists tracked middle-age and older men for 16 years. The study found that those who typically skipped breakfast were almost 30 percent more likely to have a heart attack or die from heart disease than those who regularly ate breakfast.[16] The study hypothesized that skipping breakfast unduly stressed the body.

Shortly after you wake up and before you eat, re-hydrate your body. Along with no food, you have gone many hours without any fluid intake. Your body wants and needs to drink. By quenching your thirst, you also take the edge off your hunger.[17] Also, increasing hydration increases your metabolic rate. The higher your metabolic rate, the quicker you burn calories.[18]

Another very good idea is to keep a large container of water in your fridge in which you place some slices of lemon, lime or berries. Some hotels offer this in their lobby, and it infuses the water with a very pleasant and highly palatable flavor. You can even buy special bottles or pitchers to facilitate doing this at home.

I prefer something I call "juicy water." It is a mix of about 90-95 percent water and 5-10 percent juice, usually orange juice. I drink this concoction all day long and find it especially desirable to hydrate the body after exercise. Of course, as a mixer, you can use any juice you choose. There are other excellent water flavor-boosting alternatives as well. One I love is a mix of about 50 percent seltzer water, 50 percent tap water and a splash of lemon or lime juice. It is a flavorful and lively, lightly carbonated water delight that makes drinking a lot of water much easier.

When I drink water, I prefer it well-iced. First, I simply like it better this way and find it easier to consume more when it is cold. Second, very cold water is known to help increase your metabolism even more than simple hydration alone. So, drinking icy water is beneficial.

By making your water more flavorful, you are encouraged to drink more. Keep in mind that you may think you are hungry when what you really need is to drink and quench your thirst.[19] Even if you are still hungry after drinking, it takes the edge off of your hunger, and you are likely to eat less. Water, being the lightest of all beverages, is also highly compatible with a lite lifestyle. It helps to fill you up, but it does not weigh you down emotionally or physically.

A large, filling and nutritionally satisfying breakfast leads to fewer excess calories being consumed later in the day.[20] You are less likely to give in to that 10 am snack urge. At lunchtime you are less ravenous, less likely to eat too fast or eat too much. Breakfast sets the tone for your eating pattern for the rest of the day, do not ignore it. Research backs this up. It shows that people who have lost and maintained a very significant amount of weight are much more likely to regularly eat breakfast every day than those who regain their weight over time.[21]

Nutritionally and in terms of keeping the belly full and satisfied, what constitutes a good breakfast? Many diet experts say that such a breakfast should include the following: high protein, high complex carbohydrates, good fats and high fiber.[22] Protein is filling and helps you feel full longer, so do the good fats. Complex carbs are digested much more slowly than simple carbs and sugars. They are less likely to spike your blood sugar and less likely to cause a hormonal surge that makes giving in to a mid-morning snack-attack more likely.[23] Fiber creates more bulk in your gut, which leads to a quicker feeling of satiety and causes you to consume fewer calories.[24]

The ideal mix of protein, fat and carbs varies may vary from person to person. My own perfect breakfast, which meets all of these nutritional guidelines, is the breakfast parfait. I eat it every day, although some experts suggest varying your diet from day to day. Its ingredients are the following:

- Bottom layer of low-fat, high-protein cottage cheese
- Second layer of low-sugar Greek no-fat yogurt (Greek is richer, thicker, higher protein and just feels more substantial)
- Third layer of high-fiber, whole-grain cereal
- Top layer of fruit such as berries or slivers of nuts

This concoction has it all, ample protein, lots of complex carbs and more than adequate fiber. I can attest to its staying power. Generally, it sees me through to lunch quite easily. Even at lunchtime, I am not quite as ravenous and can eat sensibly.

Snack-attack: Mid-morning and mid-afternoon

There are behaviors you can engage in to break, delay and disrupt an emotionally charged snack-attack urge. We get these urges not only when we feel hungry, but often as a response to external stress, boredom, anger, frustration and anxiety.[25] If you can, even temporarily, distract yourself from a snack-attack craving, the urge might pass without giving in to the temptation. How can you do this?

Keep in mind that the Take 5 technique provides a brief distraction and a stress reducing pause that can make a real difference. If Take 5 is not effective, you can continue with the additional panic-button steps described in Chapter 9.

On the other hand, a small, nutritionally smart snack in mid-morning and mid-afternoon is not a bad idea. Nutritionally smart means a snack that is typically nutrient-dense and high fiber, but low-fat, low-sugar and calorie light.[26] This type of snack is usually going to be a vegetable (perhaps with low-fat, low-sugar yogurt dip) or a piece of fruit. Another interesting snack, when eaten in moderation is a low-fat cheese, which is typically high in nutrients. These items have a relatively low glycemic index and convert to sugar more slowly in your body not spiking your blood sugar. It tides you over until your next significant meal. With some fullness in your belly, the edge is taken off of your hunger, and you are less likely to overeat at your next meal.

Keeping your body in a state of comfortable, very low-level fullness, where you never really allow yourself to feel ravenous, is a beneficial strategy. When you skip meals and/or deny yourself a between-meal snack, you are more likely to feel hunger pangs and pump up your emotional drive to eat and to overeat at the next meal.[27] The instincts baked into your DNA keep the desire to eat always present in your mind, and your ability to control the urge to overeat is much more difficult when you feel a high level of hunger or are feeling hangry.

Your willpower and resolve to eat sensibly is greatly reinforced with mindful and purposeful eating. It is far easier to be mindful when you construct your environment in such a way that it naturally nudges you in a direction consistent with your conscious intentions. Deliberate, mindful, healthful snacking is very brain-smart.

Lunch and Dinner

There are some very smart tactics you can take to make your lunch and dinner meal more healthful. Some of these have to do with what you eat, some with how you eat, some with the eating implements you use to serve and guide food from your plate to your mouth and some have to do with the environment in which you eat.

Taken together, these suggestions are at the core of what influences the brain to consume less food. Remember that limiting accessibility is the key to countering the instincts housed in the ancient reptilian part of your brain. Less accessibility, in its many forms and permutations, means you are very likely to eat less food and consume fewer calories by following the Whole Brain Diet Lifestyle.[28]

Pre-Meal Hydration

Before every lunch and dinner, it is very smart to speed up how quickly the belly begins to feel full (i.e., feel satiated), by doing one of the following activities. Drink one to two 8-ounce glasses of low- or no-calorie beverage.[29] Water or unsweetened tea is ideal, all natural and calorie-free. Interesting research suggests that drinking this water down in big gulps is the most effective way to do it. Apparently, drinking it down in gulps prompts the release of dopamine precipitated by quenching your thirst. This feel good dopamine encourages you to drink even more and this helps to fill the belly and bring on satiety more quickly during your meal.

Using Alcohol as a Beverage

Many people have an alcoholic beverage before dinner, with dinner or after dinner (sometimes all three). I strongly recommend that to eat smart – eat in moderation, it is highly important to limit, not necessarily eliminate, alcohol use. Alcohol powerfully, affects our being able to consume food moderately and healthfully. First, it increases your cravings for foods at the same time that it actually erodes your willpower to resist such a craving. Second, most alcoholic drinks are high-calorie with few corresponding nutritional benefits. Anything more than very moderate alcohol use is very disadvantageous to following a weight loss or dietary lifestyle modification program. It is a very good overall policy to drink as few calories as possible throughout your day.

I used to like to party, sometimes a little too much. Being in a venue with free flowing alcohol and enjoying good times and fun company, greatly lowered my inhibitions and significantly increased my imbibing. Being a naturally shy person, I found that alcohol was a wonderful, social interaction lubricant that eased my tension and awkwardness at social events.

Some years back, while partying, my over-indulgence in drink got me into trouble with my wife. It seems I was too loud and was monopolizing the conversation in what she described as a "braggadocios" manner. In fact, I was talking about myself and how proud I was of having persevered and continued to work on this book. This made my wife uncomfortable and, in no uncertain terms, she let me know of her displeasure. Right then I resolved to try and avoid such alcohol infused behavior in the future. My evolving Whole Brain Diet Lifestyle provided me with the solution. I recently developed the Take 5 technique and realized it was perfect to address this problem.

I made a commitment to myself that at the next party I would employ a Take 5, 5-minute pause, to consider whether or not taking another drink was advisable. So, at the next party, after my second drink of the evening, while considering having a third, I told myself, "Ken, Take 5." I paused and asked myself, do you really want another drink, is it a wise and prudent thing to do? This simple act, which I now use at every affair where alcohol is served, has not only spared me any further possible embarrassing activity, it has also serendipitously saved me from consuming hundreds of empty, unnecessary calories. Take 5 broke the emotional impulse and disrupted the momentum driving something that I consciously knew was not in my best interest.

The Meal

As with breakfast, a mix of protein, complex carbs, good fats and some fiber is a good option. These are nutritionally smart foods, and they contribute to more rapid feelings of fullness that signal the brain to stop eating. Another very good rule of thumb is to stop eating before you feel completely full.[30] It is likely that your brain has not yet caught up to your food intake and may feel completely full in a few minutes. Getting used to your belly not feeling totally full is brain-smart behavior. Obviously, if you stop eating at this point, you are less likely to eat too much. Always leaving at least a little bit of food on your plate may help, or you can consciously put less on your plate to begin with. Any leftover foods can easily be wrapped up for later.

Knowing when you are getting full takes some practice. You must nurture your sense of body awareness, which is an aspect of your overall sense of self-awareness. While you are developing the ability to accurately judge how full you are, simply stop eating and Take 5 once or twice during the meal, pause briefly for a few minutes and then assess how full your stomach feels. You will judge how full you are feeling with very little conscious effort. To stop eating when you are feeling merely satisfied, not completely full, becomes very natural.

Is High Variety in Your Meals, Day-to-Day Good or Bad?
Experiencing satiety has both a fundamental physical aspect and a psychological component. If you can learn how to enhance the latter, you can experience satiety more rapidly, and therefore feel full sooner, eat less food and thereby overeat less often.

Accomplishing this can present a challenge. On one hand, variety in your diet is healthful to provide an array of nutrients. On the other hand, it naturally stimulates your appetite. A balance must be struck.

If you choose to eat virtually the same breakfast and the same lunch every day, you will become bored. While this sounds like a negative, it is not, as this boredom is a powerful aid to your naturally feeling less hungry and reaching a state of satiety much more quickly. When you eat a meal with many different kinds of food that varies day-to-day, you stimulate your brain's reward center to want more and more. This is one reason why even after a big meal, you may always feel there is "room" for dessert. The idea of consuming a completely new food at the end of your meal, especially a sweet treat, is appealing to your brain, even overruling the fullness in your stomach. Eating the same breakfast and the same lunch each day is less rewarding to your brain and hastens feelings of satiation. Hence, you eat less.

You do not need to, nor should you, eat the exact same meal every day. Instead, you can choose to follow this course for a period of one month at a time and then change over to a new limited menu. When you understand and accept how this behavior is beneficial to your goal of dietary transformation and weight loss, it becomes easier to adopt and stick with it.

How Fast You Eat Your Food
How you eat and the speed with which you consume your food is critical. You want to eat slowly to give your body time to signal your brain that satiety is reached, or is close to being reached.[31] Research and common sense suggests eating more slowly leads to the intake of fewer calories. It also allows you to eat more mindfully. Eating slowly allows you to better enjoy and savor what you consume. Eat and run is not only a cliché, it is not brain-smart, as it promotes overeating.

There are many ways you can slow down the eating process and increase the amount of time you take to complete your meal:[32]

- Chew and savor your food thoroughly and slowly, observe your own chewing and force yourself to slow down.
- Put your fork or spoon down in between bites.
- Listen to a piece of music or a CD of known length, and make sure your meal continues while the music plays.

Prior to the Whole Brain Diet Lifestyle eating too fast was my undoing and caused me to overeat. I have had a lifelong "love affair" with spaghetti covered with a thick layer of meat sauce. You can have your steak or lobster, just give me a heaping plate of hot spaghetti any day. My obsession with spaghetti started early, as it was one of my Mother's best and favorite dishes. But the ultimate emotional connection for me was that it was the very first meal my future wife prepared for me and I thought it was the most delicious meal ever (although my perception may have been colored by love). Every time I eat it, it reconnects me to this nostalgic moment in my life.

My wife's spaghetti with meat sauce is high in sugar, high in fat and subsequently very high in calories. Of course, eaten occasionally and in moderation, any food, including spaghetti is not a problem. The problem for me was that I could never eat it in moderation. When faced with a teeming, hot plate of savory spaghetti my only thought was to finish it quickly so I could get more. Unfortunately, I never allowed enough time to reach satiety and I always overate.

Spaghetti is still one of my favorite meals, but now using the Whole Brain Diet Lifestyle and the Take 5 technique saves me from my gluttony. An integral part of this lifestyle focuses on eating slowly and controlling portion size. So now I do not fill my plate to occupy every square inch of available space until the plate is overflowing. Equally important, I now always eat spaghetti slowly and mindfully to maximize the taste sensation and savor every bite.

The real savior for me is using the Take 5 technique. Midway during my spaghetti meal I employ a Take 5 break to simply pause to feel how full my belly is becoming and allow time for satiety to emerge. As I approach finishing my first plate, I again Take 5 to assess if I have reached a state of comfortable fullness, of satisfaction, without being over-stuffed. I ask myself, *Ken, how are you feeling, isn't your belly full enough?* Doing this allows me to blunt any urge or cravings for a second helping, a helping that I consciously know I do not really need. The Whole Brain Diet Lifestyle powered by Take 5 has let me have my "cake" (i.e. spaghetti) and eat it too.

Eating Tools and Implements
There is scattered research pertaining to the impact of your eating tools and implements on food consumption. Let's take each eating tool and implement and discuss them separately.

Plates, Bowls and Glasses
It is well known that most people are conditioned to eating the entire portion on their plate (remember your mother's stern admonishment that there are "starving children in China who would love to have the food on your plate").[33] Portion size and portion control are of paramount importance. Use smaller plates, bowls and glasses than you traditionally use.[34] This forces you to make a conscious and mindful decision to get seconds.

Size also really matters for another important reason. The brain can be fooled, even if you know the trick in advance. If you fill an 8-inch plate with food rather than fill a 12-inch plate two-thirds full, you will likely feel fuller when eating off the 8-inch plate. This is also true for a glass whether filled with milk, a soda or any other beverage. If you completely fill a 6-ounce glass, rather than fill a 12-ounce glass half full, you feel like you have consumed more after emptying the 6-ounce glass. Why? The brain is tricked into thinking that a completely full, smaller vessel holds more than a half-full, larger vessel, even when they hold the exact same amount of food or beverage.[35]

This is also an area where heaviness actually promotes liteness in eating. When you add food to plates using dishes and glasses that are heavier than normal, you are likely to fill them with less, as it feels like you are holding a greater quantity of food or beverage than you really are. This illusion leads you to take and eat less food (for more on this phenomena see Chapter 17 on "Embodied Cognition.")

Other aspects of your plates and glasses can also make a meaningful difference. For example, it may be best to have a plate that is divided into three equal parts. One can hold the main entrée and the other two vegetables. This helps to constrain the size of the entree, usually the highest-fat and -calorie item on the plate and, at the same time, remind you to take an ample helping of high-nutrition, low-sugar, low-calorie vegetables at every meal.

There is research that indicates that contrasting the color of your plate, bowl or tablecloth with your food, influences how much eat.[36] In cases, where your food is anything but the color red, red is an excellent choice to accentuate the contrast. However, if you were eating a plate of spaghetti with marinara sauce, then a white or blue plate is ideal.

Choosing a red color is also a good choice, because the color red is universally associated with stopping or slowing down. Red color plates naturally slow down your reflexes and slow down the speed with which you consume your meals (more on this in Chapter 17 on "Embodied Cognition").

When you stop at a red light, you aren't stopping because you hear the word "stop." Rather, you automatically connect the color red with the word in a symbolic fashion.[37] Similarly, when you eat from a red-colored plate, you automatically slow down the pace in which you eat and likely eat less food overall as a consequence.

Serving Utensils, Forks, Knives and Spoons
The implements you use to serve and eat, i.e. serving utensils, forks, knives and spoons, can also make a difference in your eating style and food intake speed and quantity. You might even try your hand at chop sticks. Use smaller than typical utensils, because it lowers the likelihood of your taking an overly and unnecessarily large portion. Heavier than average weight utensils are also good. These characteristics naturally aid in slowing down your eating speed, allow you to feel like you are eating more and subsequently reduce your tendency to overeat.

Regardless of utensil size, shape or weight, put down your fork or spoon between every bite of food you take. This allows you to better focus on and savor your food, prompting you to be more mindful of your eating, to chew more thoroughly and prevent "assembly line" eating. Another useful piece of advice is to cut up your food into tiny, bite size pieces. Together, these actions obviously slow down your eating speed, which gives you time to actually experience satiety, likely before you have overeaten.

Handedness and Eating Speed
You are probably very accustomed to using your primary hand for most everyday activities, including eating. But, if you deliberately force yourself to eat with your non-primary hand, this automatically slows down your food intake.[38] You cannot use a knife or coordinate the hand-to-mouth maneuver as quickly with your opposite hand. Try it. It may be awkward at first, but you can handle it.

Another useful, yet challenging, tip is using your non-dominant hand to eat. This promotes neurogenesis and brain rewiring that can help you to further establish the new routines, break old habits, and alter your dietary lifestyle.

Creating a "Distraction-Free Zone"
Consciously construct your eating environment to be a distraction-free zone. A venue where there are as few distractions as possible from your mealtime mission of totally mindful eating. If the environment you eat in is uncomfortable in any way, in its physicality or its ambience, you will use some of your mind to attend to these distractions and take away from

concentrating on your eating experience. You do not want to actively engage your senses by watching TV, listening to some forms of radio (e.g. talk shows, rap, and high-voltage rock & roll), reading a newspaper or book or even by daydreaming.

Before you start to eat, repeat to yourself a statement like, "(*Your Name*) is going to focus intently on what he/she eats, eat slowly and savor every bite." This is a simple prep to alert your mind to the task of eating mindfully and being fully aware of the moment. You can bring the act of eating into a more fully conscious state from the semi-mindless activity you are likely accustomed to.

How about eating with other people? To deny this pleasure would be both unrealistic and unpleasant. Instead, strive to eat with like-minded people, who are not only lite in being and spirit, but who understand your desire (and hopefully it is theirs as well) to eat mindfully. I recommend you converse primarily during conversation breaks when you both or all take a pause from eating. This also help to slows down your eating pace (and serendipitously allow you to really engage with and listen to them). When you resume eating, again focus intently and mindfully on eating, away from the natural distraction of listening and engaging others in conversation. This practice takes some time to get used to and is not always feasible to implement. Changing your eating lifestyle is not always easy, but it is important, and the long-term benefits make it worth trying to change.

Where you eat, the environmental conditions in which you eat, and the chairs and tables you use also play a role in promoting a highly mindful, Whole Brain Diet Lifestyle. The chair should allow you to sit comfortably for the entire length of your meal. The chair and table should also be configured to allow you to sit close to the table and not have to reach too far or bend over in an uncomfortable manner. This makes it much easier for you to spend enough time to eat your meal slowly. At the same time, the table should be high enough to allow you to reach it easily. You want to create an environment that is conducive to lingering over your meal, giving your body plenty of time to signal your brain that it has reached a state of fullness or is at least approaching that point.

The ambient temperature and humidity play a part in the eating process as well. If it is too cold, hot, or muggy you tend to eat more quickly, probably too quickly. A comfortable climate promotes an eating speed that is most compatible with eating slowly and more mindfully. How your bodily sensations affect your attitudes, perceptions and your behavior is covered in Chapter 17 on "Embodied Cognition."

In general, eat your meals in silence without any music, TV or radio playing (although as will be noted later in the book, music can sometimes serve a useful purpose). This promotes mindfulness and the sounds of eating, chewing and crunching add to the perception that you are eating more, bringing on a state of satiety more quickly.

There is another intriguing, perhaps odd, recommendation that may also heighten your sense of mindfulness. Namely, hang a mirror in your kitchen. Seeing your image, a concrete representation of yourself, raises your awareness and aids in making eating a more mindful experience.[41]

Timing of Your Meals
Not only is eating your meals on a fixed schedule beneficial to weight control, but also time of day is important. Research on circadian body rhythms indicates that eating a very large meal at breakfast may have significantly less effect on body weight than eating it at dinnertime. In one weight loss study, early eaters lost 25 percent more weight than late eaters.[40] The implication is that our culturally influenced sequence of meal size, from very small breakfast to very large dinner, should be reversed.

It is very brain-smart to pre-plan your meals at the same time every day. By eating at pre-determined times, you train your brain to expect this to happen and instill an expectation that no matter how hungry you may feel, you will be able to eat in a few hours. This allows your brain to generate fewer emotional impulses to eat at unplanned times.[42] This presents another excellent sustaining technique that minimizes depletion of your mental energy and sustains your willpower and self-control (and reduces your likelihood of becoming hangry).

Eating Meals Out
Most of us eat some meals out and some of us, due to business needs or for other reasons, eat many meals out in a typical week. Eating out creates some special issues that need to be addressed to implement a Whole Brain Diet Lifestyle. Eating out presents a challenge to control and counter your

emotional impulses in an environment in which using common sense is much more difficult.

Eating out is expensive, so it is much harder to resist eating the complete portion put onto our plates. We hate to waste food or to seemingly waste money. Further, it is difficult to resist the freebies that come with the meal like unlimited bread and rolls. And if dessert comes with your meal, it's ever so tempting to indulge. How can you counter some of the temptations of eating out?[43]

- Tell the waiter upfront to skip the bread and rolls.
- Order, when possible, ala carte, so dessert is not included.
- Ask the waiter to bring you a doggie bag/box with your meal before you are finished, to encourage not cleaning your plate.
- When ordering a salad, ask for the dressing on the side.
- Skip any fried foods, including vegetables.
- Where allowed, consider ordering from the kiddie menu, which provides you with a smaller portion and saves you money.
- Consider ordering two appetizers when combined they are lower in calories than the complete meal.
- Eat out less often to save calories and money.

At the end of your meal and before you make a decision about ordering dessert, always Take 5. This gives you another opportunity to let satiety set in and for you to sense just how full your belly really feels. Very likely, you will decide that you do not really need or want to eat dessert. (Another tip: Do not even look at the dessert menu. Avoidance of temptation is always effective.)

There is another worthwhile tactic to use when you are eating out where there will be lots of available food. Consume a smart snack beforehand to take the edge off your hunger. You should never skip a meal in anticipation of going out.[44] Skipping a meal is too likely to unleash your animal spirits, prompting you to significantly overeat to quash your ravenous hunger.

Many of us have to contend with the special issues built into eating meals out in a restaurant. With common sense, judgment and discretion you can deal with most of these issues. You can still enjoy and look forward to eating out, but using the guidelines you can do so while more easily adhering to the Whole Brain Diet Lifestyle.

Eating After Dinner

Making dinner the last time you eat makes good sense. In addition to not consuming any additional calories, your body needs four to five hours after your last food consumption to fire up your metabolic furnace and prepare the body for fat and calorie burning.[45] If you eat later in the evening, you delay the onset of this activity and limit the fat-burning and calorie depletion part of your day. Also, if you go to sleep on a stomach that is fairly full, you may have difficulty staying asleep.

I always found the temptation to snack especially alluring during my post dinner, wind-down period, an activity many people engage in nightly. There was a time when I, as many others do, watched TV in the evening while munching on junk food. Tired and distracted from watching the "boob tube," this eating was typically mindless with only limited awareness of how much I was actually consuming. One night, after a round of particularly mindless snacking, I realized I had eaten a whole bag of Cheetos and I resolved to do better. This occurred in the early days of my development of the Whole Brain Diet Lifestyle when I was coming to the realization, based on my research, that willpower grows weaker during the day as we tire. I realized that by 8pm, my willpower and resolve to snack sensibly was greatly diminished.

I needed a plan to counter this normal daily occurrence and I found it. A key premise of the Whole Brain Diet Lifestyle plan is that our brain craves certainty and routine. I came to the realization that the most effective way to end mindless TV snacking is to eliminate it entirely. Since that time, when tempted to have a snack, or eat anything after dinner, I simply say to myself, "Ken chooses to not eat anything after dinner." This simple ploy provides my brain with a certainty it finds reassuring and avoids a nightly decision on whether to snack or not. No decision is required as it was pre-made, so there is no need to depend on willpower to avoid yielding to temptation. Sometimes an absolute, inviolable rule is the best one. Since I instilled this rule my nighttime snacking (excluding parties or other social occasions) has gone to zero and yours can too.

Instilling a general rule that you do not eat after dinner simplifies your life and your decision making. You do not need to make a daily decision as to whether or not to have a snack after dinner, since the decision is already made. As with all sustaining actions, this one conserves your mental energy, minimizes its depletion and helps to sustain your willpower and self-control.

Another simple tip discourages eating after dinner, and reinforces your absolute, no post dinner snacking rule, is to brush your teeth shortly after finishing your dinner.[46] This provides a cue to yourself that you are not planning on eating any more that evening. Another tip is to turn off your kitchen lights as a symbol and sign to your brain that the kitchen and your eating is finished for the day.

Similar to my need to control nighttime snacking in front of the TV, a few years ago I found that I was surreptitiously slipping into a pattern of having a glass of wine during the day, in mid-afternoon. I usually listen and relax to music every day at this time and a glass of wine seemed to fit into the experience and ambience I was trying to create. I was long accustomed to having a glass of wine in the evening after dinner. But I was leery and uncomfortable at the prospect of establishing a daytime ritual that involved drinking alcohol, as there is a history of alcohol abuse in my immediate family.

I resolved to not let this become a routine and to stop this practice before it took hold. I found a highly effective solution by employing the same tool that I used to stop my post-dinner snacking. As my daytime wine drinking routine was not yet well established, I was able to stop it cold, by making an absolute pledge to myself and saying, "Ken chooses to not ever drink alcohol before 5pm." This leaves no wiggle room for interpretation or being able to rationalize an excuse as to why I could make an exception just this time. This mantra works extremely well for me.

Part of the Whole Brain Diet Lifestyle is firmly grounded on some understanding of human behavior and human decision-making practices. Your unconscious self sometimes guides you to make a choice that you desire (like enjoying a daytime glass of wine), which your conscious self knows is not a good, healthy choice and should be avoided. Giving your brain a measure of constancy and certainty makes your brain happy and a happy brain puts you in a better position to make choices based on doing what you consciously know is the right thing to do, e.g., not drinking alcohol in the daytime. It all goes back to the central core mantra of the Whole

Brain Diet Lifestyle, "Your brain is the master of your behavior and YOU are the master of your brain."

Creating Conscious Intentions

Using the principles I utilized throughout my career in consumer research, advertising and marketing, I know that one approach to effectively communicating and reinforcing a message is to use a repetitive saturation campaign. In this context, set up your physical environment in a way that constantly exposes you to psychological messages that promote your goal of realizing significant changes to your dietary lifestyle.

In all the places where you spend time and where you normally consume foods and snacks, you want to see statements, sayings and symbols that promote, eat smart – eat in moderation and promote using the Take 5 technique. Specifically, in your house, your kitchen, by your TV, in your car, in your office and at a restaurant, you want to always be able to see a message that promotes the changes you are trying to achieve.

This includes some of the previous alerts and reminders discussed, such as the Fat Bottle in your kitchen and by your TV; the big pointing NO finger affixed to your snack cabinet/drawer; and, the Take 5 wristband I recommend you wear at all times. Additionally, I recommend that you consider the following:

- Refrigerator magnets placed by the door handle of your 'fridge with messages such as:
    - Eat smart – eat in moderation
    - Take 5
    - Sugar Can Be Toxic
    - Delay Gratification Now-Lose Weight Later
    - *Fat* brain – *Skinny* brain: I Choose to Follow My *Skinny* Brain
- Self-adhesive stickies for your mirrors and glass surfaces with messages such as those above
- A clip-on tag for your inside car mirror with similar messages
- A plaque for your office desk urging you to eat smart – eat in moderation or to Take 5

The goal is to present these messages wherever you are and whenever you might be tempted to eat in excess or otherwise eat inappropriately. By this means, you create messages for yourself that permeate your psyche. Once created and internalized, these messages act to build and to maintain your mental energy and hence your willpower and resolve to follow a new dietary lifestyle.

Increasing Availability to Healthful Foods

Construct your environment to make sure that you always have ready access to low-sugar, low-calorie foods to help and encourage you to choose a healthy alternative when you are ready to snack. This means having these healthy snacks always within reach at home or at work.

Growing up, my parents always kept vegetables like carrots and celery sticks cut-up in cold water in the fridge. When a snack-attack did emerge, there was always a healthy alternative within arm's reach. Most offices also have a fridge available where such a snack could be stored and easily retrieved each workday.

Keeping fresh fruits such as cherries and apples in a highly visible and accessible location, is also very smart. Not only are they relatively low on the glycemic index, their natural sugar can help to satisfy your sweet tooth as well. Remember that your brain craves sugar, and sugar found naturally in food is far healthier than consuming food containing a lot of refined sugar.

The point is not that you always make a low-calorie snack choice, but that you will do so much more often when a healthy alternative is readily within your view and reach.

The Workplace

Your office environment, where many of you spend eight hours per day or longer, is often a snacking paradise. Snacks are often accessible, often right on your own desk or that of a nearby colleague. A study conducted by the University of Illinois showed that merely putting candy in an opaque bowl, rather than a clear bowl, reduced consumption by 40 percent.[47] You may not be able to influence your office mates to remove the snacks from the office, but you can certainly do so for your own desk and immediate surroundings or at least make them seem less accessible.

Thanksgiving and Beyond: The Perils of the Holiday Season

The entire holiday season, from Thanksgiving through New Year's and maybe even through Super Bowl Sunday, is filled with occasions where you are encouraged by societal norms, family and friends, to eat, drink and be merry. For those of you concerned about your weight, it is a perilous time of year. The whole tenor and mood of the holiday season is to let your inhibitions go, to let your guard down and to have fun. As a result, you are very likely to weigh more on the second of January than any other day of year. The ensuing winter season is when your body enters a natural state of fat accumulation. Since the weather and less daylight hours discourage outside exercise, nature conspires to make winter weight gain likely and winter weight loss very, very difficult. If you gain just two to three pounds over the holidays, in just 10 years you can gain considerable weight.[48]

The holiday season is fraught with challenges. The access to an abundance of free food and alcohol is a huge trigger event prompting overeating and over-drinking. To begin, before each prime occasion where overeating and/or over-drinking is likely, repeat to yourself the following statement:

"(Your Name) knows that today presents a special eating challenge, but he/she chooses, and pledges that he/she will still eat (and drink) smart and in moderation and always Take 5."

You can also employ the following tactics. The day or two before a holiday event, you can consciously moderately reduce your caloric intake and increase your physical activity. On the day of the social occasion, just like the advice I gave to not skip breakfast, do not completely skip a meal as a counter measure. This makes overeating far more likely.

If you are with your partner, try to boost your intent and resolve to eat smart - eat in moderation. Ask them to give you a pre-arranged signal, innocuous to others but observable by you, if they see you overindulging in food or drink. Just having such an arrangement, even if never employed, makes you more mindful about the amount you are consuming. If your partner gives you the signal, it may well save you hundreds of calories.

At a holiday party or social affair, eat and socialize, but not both at the same time. When you eat and talk, it is much more difficult to be highly mindful as you tend to be very distracted. It is then hard to be alert and focused on how much you are eating or drinking.

Many parties and holiday dinners are served buffet-style, and these represent an especially challenging situation. You are much more likely to take extra large portions of the foods you like from a buffet than when you are served by others. So, survey the buffet first and decide which items you most want to have. In addition, try to not fill one super-large plate with all of your food. If possible, use a small plate for the highest-calorie foods and a larger plate for the lower-calorie fruits and vegetables. Also, be mindful that even eating healthy foods like turkey can pack a lot of calories if you overfill your plate. How you eat your turkey matters. Selecting white meat over dark, removing the skin and skipping the gravy can save you from consuming a lot of unnecessary calories.

Try not to be among the last to leave the party, especially a party where alcohol and appetizers are distributed freely. The longer you stay, the higher your risk of overeating or overdrinking. As the night wears on, your inhibitions tend to be relaxed, your willpower wanes and the odds of your over-indulging skyrocket.

If you follow any, or all, of this advice, you can survive the season with minimal to no weight gain and still enjoy the holidays.

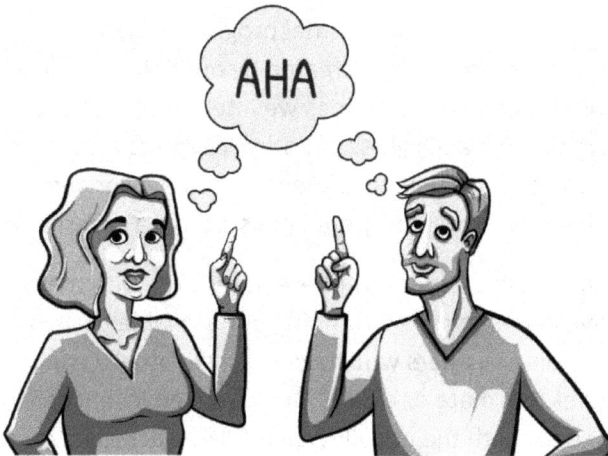

- You can consciously fool your brain into a desired response even when you know the trick ahead of time. For example, keeping unhealthy foods out of your line of vision makes you much less likely to eat them, even if in reality they are only a very short distance away. As the old adage says, out of sight, out of mind.
- Make it easier for yourself to make the healthy choice by having healthful snacks always easily accessible. All of us usually take the path of least resistance, and that path is typically the one that offers the most readily accessible snack item.

Chapter 12: Genes and Memes

Genes and memes are fundamental to the human experience but poorly understood or misunderstood by most.

This chapter was inspired and informed by two provocative books, *Super Genes*,[1] written by Rudy Tanzi and Deepak Chopra and *Virus of the Mind*,[2] written by Richard Brody.

Super Genes, elaborates on the science behind the phenomenon known as epigenetics and how our conscious and unconscious experiences effect and alter the expression and functioning of our genes. They explain that while our genes have a profound impact on our behavior and our health, they provide direction, a tendency toward an outcome, but they don't (except in very few cases) determine the outcome. We have the ability to be the user, director and guide of our genes by changing our beliefs and our lifestyle.

In *Virus of the Mind*, Richard Brody discusses the science of memetics. He says, "Memes are the building blocks of your mind, the programming of your mental computer." It starts with the premise that our fundamental behaviors are a function of our mental programming and our environment. And our mental programming is created by our DNA-bred instincts, hardwired into our brain, and the memes we internalize that encapsulate our core beliefs, attitudes and values. A critical caveat is that we can choose, consciously and deliberately, to influence our behavior and our health even when our tendency, directed by our genes, favors a different outcome.

Being overweight, and especially obese, interferes with maximizing our ability to have and enjoy sex by limiting our available partners. In particular, it limits our finding partners who have the instinctually appealing attributes most of us seek in a mate or a date. Our distorted instinct to overeat for survival is at odds with the equally powerful instinct to have sex for pleasure and procreation.

How can you resolve this dilemma? One novel way is to frequently repeat a mantra to yourself until it becomes internalized and imprinted onto your brain. In this way, these mantras morph into being similar to a traditional meme that others pass on to you via word-of-mouth or social media and "infect your mind." Except, in this case, you, consciously, act as your own "meme" propagator. You can employ these self-infused memes to help motivate you to eat smart - eat in moderation. Remember, your behavior is directed by a combination of your mental programming, based on your genes, memes and environment. By using memes, even ones you create for yourself, you quiet the impulses generated by your *Fat* brain.

Aids such as a Take 5 wristband, magnets and images are types of visual memes. There are memes that you repeat out loud, or silently, to yourself every day to reinforce the basic notion of eat smart – eat in moderation.

The first set of memes we propose are those that consciously promote the themes that being overweight or obese limits your opportunity to find an optimal mate and/or have frequent sex. These memes raise the saliency of this theme in your mind and reinforce the latent feelings you likely already possess about your weight. These include the following memes:

- Lose Weight and Gain a Mate
- Lose Weight and Find a Date
- Lose Weight and Your Sex Life Will Be Great
- Take 5 and Your Weight Will Dive

If you repeat these mantras to yourself and say them out loud (or write them in journal), every day, you can use the power of a meme to download these thoughts to your subconscious emotional self. There they can serve to counter your distorted drive to overeat. Whether you are single and searching for a mate or in a committed relationship, you can use sexually related memes to reinforce what you already likely believe to be true, i.e., excess weight is detrimental to achieving an optimal sex life.

Even when you are aware of your intent to internalize a meme in order to influence your behavior, your brain cooperates with your intentions. This is particularly true when the memes you are trying to reinforce are consistent with your pre-existing beliefs. Most of us believe that being overweight reduces one's attractiveness and makes us less appealing to others, so most of us readily accept them as valid. This makes them easier to incorporate into your unconscious self and more powerful in their impact on your behavior.

I also propose a second set of memes that directly promote a healthy dietary lifestyle, one that is brain-smart, nutritionally wise and furthers your goal to eat smart – eat in moderation. Note that these memes are all stated in the third person, starting with your name, instead of "I" will, it says you, (i.e., YOUR NAME) will do something. As previously mentioned, stating an intention in the third person, not in the first person, strengthens the intention and makes it even more powerful in its ability to influence your behavior.

These memes include:

- (*Your Name*) eats a high-sugar, high-carb, high-calorie dessert only on Sunday.
- (*Your Name*) always stops eating when he/she feels about three-quarters full.
- (*Your Name*) never eats anything after dinner.
- (*Your Name*) eats to live, he/she does not live to eat.
- (*Your Name*) always Takes 5 to stay alive.

These memes incorporate ideas that can be used to transform your dietary lifestyle. They are important and useful to reinforce your intentions and make achieving a dietary lifestyle change more probable. Internalizing these two sets of memes boosts your mental energy as your subconscious emotional self is in concert with your conscious self. When both parts are aligned, your mental energy is naturally boosted, and you do not need to expend as much mental energy trying to reconcile competing impulses. Exercising your self-control allows you to forgo a temptation and to be more mindful of the need to eat smart - eat in moderation.

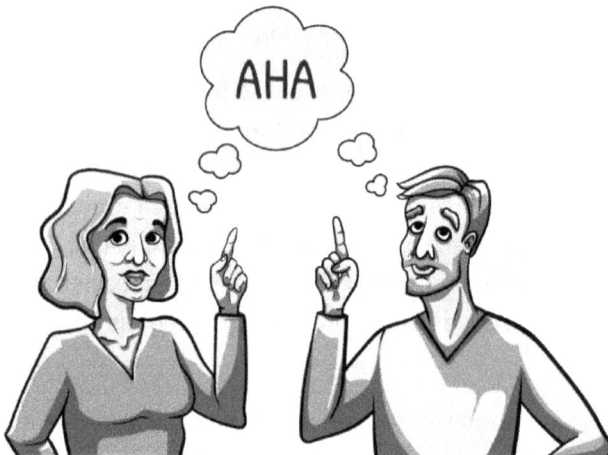

- A combination of your genes, memes and environment are instrumental in determining your behavior and health outcomes.

But, they are <u>not</u> fixed in stone, and you can use your conscious efforts and experiences to alter them to your benefit.

- Self-preservation and perpetuation of our species are the two most fundamental of your DNA-bred instincts, but you can use self-infused memes to help counter your instincts driving you to overeat and, simultaneously, strengthen your intention to eat smart – eat in moderation.

Chapter 13: Exercise

Repeat this mantra: "It's All Exercise." Make it part of your daily routine and it will change your life.

Some pundits have said that if you could capture all of the benefits of exercise and encapsulate it in one pill, people would pay an exorbitant price to take it. How ironic that you can actually enjoy a great deal of the mental, physical and spiritual benefits of exercise for virtually no cost. Some of the best forms of exercise require only a short amount of time and having a conscious intention and commitment to regularly engage in the activity.

Kelly Traver summarizes the benefits of exercise very well saying, "exercise is your biggest ally in health and in behavior change because it optimizes the performance of both the body and the brain."[1]

Exercise is a natural part of adopting a lite approach to life. By burning calories and releasing endorphins, it promotes and boosts a liteness of mood, spirit and body. This liteness builds your mental energy, willpower and self-control.

The Benefits of Exercise

The following list is merely a brief recitation of the multi-faceted and varied benefits associated with exercise[2]:

- Significantly reduce feelings and negative effects associated with stress.
- Increases muscle mass, burns calories and increases your metabolism to use more calories afterward.
- Creates more neural connections in the brain, creating a healthier, more alert and better memory.[3]
- Can prevent or delay the onset of dementia such as Alzheimer's disease.
- Strengthens the immune system, making us more resistant to illness and disease.
- Strengthens the cardiovascular system, making you more resistant to heart disease.
- Reduces the risk of getting some cancers.
- Increases mental alertness, refreshes the body and lessens feelings of fatigue.
- Reduces feelings of some chronic pain.

- Promotes increased bone density and strength.
- Increases your feelings of self-control and self-efficacy raising your overall feelings of well-being.

Research also shows that exercise has important effects on your mental and emotional health. Exercise not only can ameliorate the symptoms of depression, it can also help prevent it from occurring in the first place. Your overall level of fitness and your mental health are highly correlated.[4]

Exercise can play an important role in helping you to lose weight, although exercise alone is usually not enough to facilitate a large weight loss. There are no better activities that you can engage in to help optimize the performance of your brain and body. It is clear that humans today get far, far less exercise than in the early days of Homo sapiens, a few hundred years ago or even fifty years ago. This is one of the fundamental factors driving obesity in the modern world.

Thirty to sixty minutes of exercise on most days, can burn a significant number of calories by itself, and it provides benefits in other less direct ways.[5] In addition to increasing the burn rate of calories directly and then continuing to burn calories by raising your metabolism for a period of time, exercise offers other huge benefits. These include:[6]

- Help to reduce emotionally-driven urges based on feelings of loneliness, anger, frustration or boredom that cause mindless, unhealthy eating
- Increasing feelings of self-confidence, a sense of efficacy and a sense that you can really affect change in your life
- Directly lighting up your brain's reward centers via an increase in the production of neurotransmitters like serotonin and dopamine. This helps you substitute a positive desired behavior (i.e. exercise) for a negative, undesired one like overeating or inappropriate snacking

Paul Dudley White, a famed physician and healer, offers another highly substantive rationale for sustaining an exercise program, "A vigorous five-mile walk will do more good for an unhappy, but otherwise healthy adult then all the medicine and psychology in the world."[7]

Exercise is an excellent means of maximizing your willpower by renewing the mental energy that fuels your self-control. Exercise serves a dual role both to build mental energy and as an excellent sustaining tactic that mitigates stress.

Serendipitously, exercise has even another subtle benefit that aids you in your quest to transform your diet lifestyle, making it an essential and powerful aid. When you incorporate exercise into your regular, ideally daily routine, it becomes easier to make other changes as well. Once you start to take better care of yourself, it becomes pervasive, influencing other parts of your life in a virtuous cycle.

Exercise aids you in aligning your higher-order conscious intentions with your subconscious emotional self. Once accomplished, this synergistically multiples your mental energy, willpower, resolve and self-control. Your ability to live a life of moderation, to be more mindful, to eat smart – eat in moderation and to live a lite lifestyle becomes much more feasible.

While regular sustained exercise is important, even regular exercise cannot completely undo the deleterious effects on longevity from sitting for too long. Uninterrupted and prolonged sitting is corelated with premature death. Take 5 every 30 to 60 minutes to stand and move, which can undo the negative effects of sitting for a long time.[8]

How to Encourage Yourself to Start and Continue an Exercise Program

You can help to increase your will and resolve to exercise by[9]:

- Starting a new exercise program slowly, and progress at a conservative pace.
- Having a specific intent and plan to exercise, including the particular days and times you intend to do it (the brain loves stability and constancy).
- Making sure you own very comfortable, supportive and appropriate clothing, shoes and other accessories to facilitate the exercise.
- Taking advantage of opportunities to engage in physical activity when you can (e.g. park far from your destination; take the stairs; get up from your desk and take a 5-minute walk break; walk to the local store).

- Listening to music when you walk or jog, as it helps time pass in a pleasant way. However, care must be taken to be observant to your surroundings.
- Varying your walking/jogging route.
- Try to make exercise a social activity and work out with a friend.
- If you exercise long enough and over a sufficient period of time, it becomes an integral part of your life, and you actually look forward to it (i.e., exercise makes your brain happy).
- Take a day off a week to allow your body to rebuild.
- Take additional days off if you feel discomfort, pain, or prolonged fatigue. If these continue, see a doctor immediately. The old adage "No Pain, No Gain" is not true.

It does all this while simultaneously promoting better physical health by burning calories, reducing blood pressure and boosting blood flow and oxygen to the brain.

There is another interesting perspective about exercise that you can employ to increase your will, resolve and likelihood to exercise. A regular, lifelong exercise program is estimated to add three to five years to your expected longevity as well as significantly increase the quality of your life.[11]

If the pharmaceutical industry could sell you a pill that provided you with a likely benefit of five additional years to live, how much would you be willing to pay for it? You might be willing to spend $10,000, $100,000, maybe even more. All you have to do is devote a moderate number of minutes per day and hours per week to exercise, and you can have a longer life for virtually no cost. Keep this truth in mind, there is no better deal on Earth than exercise.

When you are exercising and feel your will to continue is waning, it's another excellent time to Take 5. The Take 5 five-minute pause can give you a chance to get a second breath, and a brief pause can reboot your brain for more physical activity. When combined with performing a few stretches, the body emerges from Take 5 ready for more.

Use of Rewards as an Exercise Motivator

The use of external rewards and penalties can significantly bridge the transition period between initiation of a new behavior (e.g. exercise) and its internalization as an automatic and routine practice. Once exercise becomes habit, it provides its own intrinsic rewards to your brain and body that automatically reinforce its continued usage; in the meantime, a reward program boosts your motivation to exercise.

As with weight loss or weight loss maintenance, rewards boost willpower and promote perseverance and adherence to your program. The great long-distance runner Jim Ryun once said, "Motivation is what gets you started. Habit is what keeps you going."[13] Once acquired, all habits, whether good or bad for you, are self-sustaining; you just have to reach the point where the behavior becomes automatic and routine, and using rewards can you help you to accomplish this.

For each milestone reached, like sustaining your exercise activity for a week, a month, or a quarter, you should set up, in advance, a series of rewards for accomplishing each goal.

Even on an annual basis and well into the future, you can use rewards to help reinforce your exercise routine. You could do something really special with the money you save on the health-related costs and mindless snacking you avoid. In an average year, you will realize hundreds of dollars of savings (and possibly much, much more) if you exercise regularly.

Other Activities to Motivate You to Continue to Exercise
There are a few other activities you can engage in to further reinforce and promote your continued participation in an exercise program.

- Use psychological reinforcement (pre-bed and post-awakening) by reading statements and viewing images that help you realize that you can achieve this goal and raise your expectation in your ability to do so. Statements like:
    o My brain is the master of my behavior, and I am the master of my brain.
    o Exercise optimizes my brain and my body.
    o I choose to do good things for myself, and exercise is one of those good things that I choose to do.
    o Regular exercise is very healthy for my mind and body, it saves me a lot money.
    o I choose to exercise today and every day.

- Visualize yourself as a healthier, more vibrant and more energized person.

These activities help to infuse your subconscious with your conscious intent to exercise, bringing them into a powerful alignment that strengthens your resolve to continue exercising.

Mind-set and Exercise: Reframing Your Attitudes

The most important mind-set you can have to encourage exercise is to reframe your attitude toward exercise. Like most people, I used to bristle at my wife's request to do some chore, run some errand or otherwise exert myself physically. Until one day, I had an epiphany: **"It's all exercise!"** Sounds trite, but it's true. Next time you are asked to do something, anything that requires movement, remember: It is really all exercise, and it's all good. The "it's all exercise" mantra is backed by research reported in the University of California, Berkeley, Wellness Letter, that very short periods of physical activity pay off.[14] The accumulation of very short periods of physical exertion, like for a minute or two, have the same highly beneficial effects on physical markers (e.g. cholesterol, blood pressure, blood sugar level and waist size), as much longer sustained physical activity, as long as the overall time spent on physical activity is similar.

Why Exercise Is So Natural to Humans

Early hominid species and early Homo sapiens relied on strenuous physical activity to maximize their odds for survival. Hunter-gatherers who did not tolerate a high level of physical exertion or could not quickly flee a predator or a foe were less likely to survive to the age of reproduction. Evolution favored those who were good at high physical activity that could be sustained for the extended period of time needed to wear down an animal food source, find a scarce natural food or flee a predator.

The need to move, to exert ourselves, to exercise, is built into our evolutionary history. That is why humans are natural exercising machines. But in the era of hunter-gatherers, energy expenditure may have been skewed, with long intense periods of great physical exertion followed by extended periods of rest and non-physical activity. People hunted and gathered food, ate, rested and slept. Life was much simpler and less complex.

In today's world, we do not need such extended periods of intense physical activity to survive nor, do many of us, have the time to indulge in very long periods of non-sleep rest.[15] All physical exertion stokes your metabolism and increases your rate of burning calories. So, when my wife asks me to do a chore, I try to recall that simple, motivating truth: *It's all exercise.* Remember, all movement and activities that you may not typically perceive as exercise can be viewed through a different and more positive lens.

How Much Exercise Do You Need?

The experts generally recommend that you exercise a minimum 150 minutes per week, which might translate in to 30 minutes five days per week or some other combination. But most exercise physiologists believe that more is even better. For example, engaging in about 250 minutes per week is excellent and as much as 450 minutes per week is ideal. But, even as little as 15 minutes per day of moderate exercise can reduce your risk of dying prematurely.[16]

I personally walk on average six to seven days per week for 60 to 90 minutes per day, or a total of around seven to ten hours per week. Rarely do I have 90 minutes straight to walk, so I break my walks up into a morning and afternoon session. Not everyone has this much time to devote to a planned exercise program, but having a goal that stretches you a bit is beneficial and helps you to do more.

You should, however, keep in mind the wisdom of the old adage, "Everything in moderation." Exercise as a weight loss aid is best when conducted consistently, at a moderate level of intensity. If you engage frequently in extreme activity, you are more likely to reward yourself with food, because your body craves it, and you may subconsciously feel that you have "earned it."

There is also evidence suggesting that while moderate, sustained exercise acts as an appetite suppressant, intense prolonged exercise stimulates your appetite. Maintaining balance in your life is a brain-smart way of living, applicable to exercise as well as being an excellent overall philosophy for life.

Where You Exercise

How much you exercise is important, but also important is where you choose to exercise. Research suggests that exercising outdoors is more beneficial than exercising indoors on several dimensions that benefit both the body and the brain.[17]

Exercise benefits your brain, mind and spirit. Research indicates that being in a natural setting, outside among the trees, plants, flowers and streams on a sunny day makes your brain happy.[18] The potential problems of the weather notwithstanding, exercising outdoors is simply better and more enjoyable than exercising indoors.

Being outdoors releases feel-good neurotransmitters that act to reinforce your exercise routine and make it more likely that you continue it. Mankind evolved in the outdoors before there were any shelters. Being in the sun is totally natural to us, and that is why it feels so good. If you are unable to exercise daily, try to pick those days when the sun shines, and utilize the power of the sun to enhance your mental energy, to reduce stress and to make you feel good, all of which will help to reinforce your exercise routine.

When You Exercise

When you exercise is quite important. Specifically, exercising early in the morning is ideal for several reasons. First, your mental energy (and hence your willpower and motivation) peaks early in the day. This makes getting out early to exercise less burdensome and more natural. Second, once you are done, you can begin to enjoy the daily benefits of exercising right away, and if so inclined, enjoy some more of it later in the day.

There is another significant rationale as well. When you exercise, you need energy, i.e. you must expend calories, to fuel your activity. If you exercise early in the day and before you eat breakfast your body is more likely to burn stored fat than the more readily accessible sugars that you consume at breakfast.[19]

Listening to Your Body

Keep in mind that exercise can be both self-correcting and self-reinforcing. If you overdo it, exercise too hard or for too long, you will likely get tired, sore and injured. This should encourage you to ease off, slow down and heal and therefore lose your exercise rhythm. Listen to your body. If you don't, you will be much less likely to continue your exercise routine over the long-run.

At the same time, exercise can be self-reinforcing. If you engage in a regular exercise program for a long enough time, you will eagerly anticipate going out and exercising, enjoy the exercise time itself, and feel positive emotions and increased well-being after each round of exercise.

Exercise alone is not a complete prescription for weight loss. Yet it is useful to help you lose weight and especially useful to help sustain a weight loss.

Walking and Working: Perfect Together
There is a myth in American business still perpetuated today that is incorrect. The myth is that a good metric for measuring work output is the number of hours a worker spends on the job, in the office. For far too many employers, time spent in the office at one's desk is still used as a proxy to assess if the employee is being productive. Total time spent in the office is not highly correlated with measuring real productive output.

I speak from personal experience based on observations of hundreds of employees over an almost forty-year career. For part of my career, I worked for a man who figuratively, if not literally, counted the number of minutes his employees were seated at their desk as productive time, and all else as non-productive. If I had suggested that taking a walking break during office hours could and likely would have boosted my total productivity, he would have laughed me off as being ridiculous. But that is exactly what I am proposing to you and your employer.

Employers should encourage their employees to take a 10- to 15-minute walk outdoors at least once per day and ideally twice a day. The result is a meaningful improvement in the quality and creativity of employee work output and likely the quantity as well.

Any physical movement, but especially rhythmic movement like walking, particularly in an outdoors setting, provides many benefits. Stress, mental strain and fatigue are the enemies of motivation, willpower and creative thinking. You cannot simply use your determination to disrupt a mental block or work through a seemingly intractable, complex problem. Movement frees up the brain, declutters the mind, refocuses your concentration and recharges your willpower and motivation.

A ten- to fifteen-minute walk outdoors has all of the following additional benefits:

- Promotes problem-solving by quieting a noisy brain.
- Facilitates creative thinking and brainstorming.
- Defuses boredom and frustration that undermine productive thinking.
- Increases one's stamina to see a task through to completion.

Taking a walk provides an excellent interlude to engage in alone or with a colleague or even your boss. One of my favorite managers often invited me outside to walk and talk through difficult topics and problems. These problems were usually directly work based, but sometimes more personally related. No matter what their nature, walking and talking helped to solve or resolve them more quickly, more effectively and much more pleasantly then in an office across a desk from one another.

Research on the impact of walking at work on walkers' immediate mood and energy concluded, "On the afternoons after a lunchtime stroll, walkers said they felt considerably more enthusiastic, less tense, and generally more relaxed and able to cope than on afternoons when they hadn't walked and even compared with their own moods from a morning before a walk."[17] These are emotional states that are highly associated not only with better morale and happier employees, but also higher productivity.

How does this all relate to adopting a brain-smart and healthy lifestyle? You may recall what Kelly Traver says in her book about exercise optimizing both the body and the brain for peak performance. Further, and more directly relevant to adopting a Whole Brain Diet Lifestyle, the proverbial 10 am and 3 pm snack-attack can be deterred and replaced by an equally satisfying and energizing walk. Not only are unnecessary calories not consumed, but additional calories are expended in the process.

Steve Jobs was one of the most visionary American entrepreneurs. He was also well-known for incorporating walking and talking into his business practices alone and with employees who worked for him and others who wished to work with him. He demonstrated that walking and working were actually perfect together.

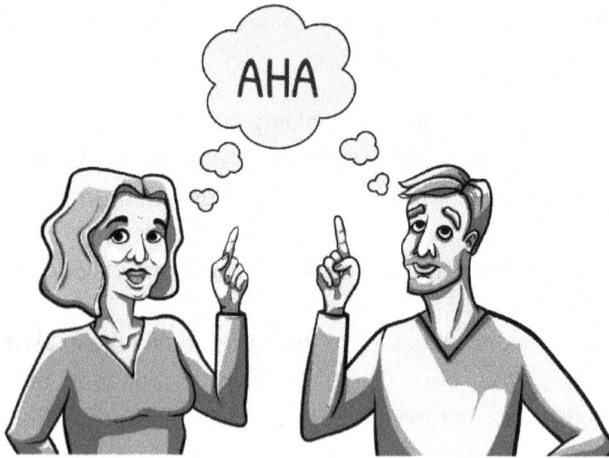

- Regular exercise is the single best activity you can do for your heart and for your brain and to facilitate neuronal growth that makes behavioral change more likely. Exercise is closer to a magic bullet for the health of your body and brain than any other alternative. Perhaps if you could <u>not</u> do it for free, you would better appreciate its awesome value and its ability to fundamentally improve your life and your well-being.
- Physical exertion and exercise are strongly favored by evolution and makes your brain very, very happy. Give exercise a chance to become routine, and you likely will look forward to it every day-just like I do.

Chapter 14: Stress

Minor stress is energizing and productive; acute stress arms the body against a threat; but chronic stress simply corrodes the body and mind.

What Is Stress?

Stress can be identified and experienced as a sudden surge of adrenaline when you perceive a potential threat to your safety and well-being. This could be spotting a snake or wild animal, hearing a sound in your house late at night, seeing a strange person walking toward you on a lonely street or any other unexpected stimuli.

The stress reaction arms the body and the mind readying it to take an immediate action to preserve your survival and well-being via a fight or flight response. Without such a stress-induced response, you would be much more vulnerable to attack from a predatory animal, person or other potentially existential threat. Stress makes you feel alert, focused, strong and energetic, which could save your life if faced with a real physical threat.

However, like so many other mind-body states or behaviors, there is a delicate balance between feeling too much and too little stress. There is an optimal level that varies from person to person that is good, healthy and life-preserving, but a chronically high level of stress is dangerous to your life and well-being.

Stress Related Symptoms and Problems

Negative warning signs and symptoms of too much stress include the following[1].

Cognitive Symptoms

Memory problems
Inability to concentrate
Poor judgment
Seeing only the negative
Anxious or racing thoughts
Constant worrying

Emotional Symptoms

Moodiness
Irritability or short temper
Agitation, inability to relax
Feeling overwhelmed
Sense of loneliness
Depression or unhappiness

Physical Symptoms	Behavioral Symptoms
Aches and pains	Eating more or less
Diarrhea or constipation	Sleeping too much or too little
Nausea, dizziness	Isolating yourself from others
Chest pain, rapid heartbeat	Procrastinating
Loss of sex drive	Using alcohol/cigarettes/drugs
Frequent colds	Nervous habits

Chronic stresses can also lead to very serious and debilitating health effects such as:

- Heightened sensitivity to pain
- Heart disease
- Muscle ache
- Chronic headaches
- Depression
- Sleep disorders
- Overeating and inappropriate snacking
- Increased likelihood of experiencing Alzheimer's disease
- More rapid aging of the mind and body

Another highly damaging effect of chronic stress is its impact on cellular inflammation, a danger unknown to many people. Mild and transient inflammation is beneficial in moderation and when needed to fight infection. But it is potentially deadly when chronic. Inflammation is thought by some medical research experts to be a highly important, independent risk factor and a primary cause of heart disease and other chronic ailments.

Inflammation is also now identified as an important facilitating factor in the progression of Alzheimer's by speeding the death of brain cells and promoting a negative feedback loop that escalates the rate of disease progression. Controlling and reducing inflammation through stress mitigation is a highly brain-smart activity.

How Stress Can Affect Overeating and Weight Gain

There are multiple ways in which experiencing stress can affect your likelihood to overeat and gain weight. These include[2]:

- triggering hunger hormones that drive overeating

- increased cravings for foods high in carbs and sugar
- depressing your metabolic rate, causing you to burn calories more slowly
- disrupting your sleep
- feeling extra time pressure that prompts you to skip a meal and overeat later in the day

Adopting the Whole Brain Diet Lifestyle reduces your perception of stress and mitigates its effects when experienced. It aids you significantly in controlling overeating and nutritionally poor eating but also reduces the negative effects of stress on the inflammation response.

How does stress affect your diet lifestyle? Specifically, stress can severely deplete your willpower and make it difficult to renew your resolve that enables you to resist inappropriate food choices and unplanned snacking.[3]

Ways in Which You Can Reduce Stress

As Kelly Traver says in her book *The Program: The Brain-Smart Approach to the Healthiest You*, stress is a physiologic response to an event, not the event itself. If stress is a mental phenomenon, before it is physically manifested, you can use your brain to manage and minimize its negative consequences.

One great and quick way to mitigate the effects of stress and minimize its impact on your mind-body is to employ the Take 5 technique. Breathing rhythmically and deeply in and out can reduce the momentum of a stressor. The more you practice Take 5 to disarm a craving to eat or drink unhealthfully, the more you can readily employ it to quickly disrupt a stress response.

Some of the best known and most trusted ways to reduce stress include engaging in the following behaviors:[4]

- regular exercise
- progressive muscle relaxation
- getting adequate sleep
- using meditation
- listening to music
- eating a well-balanced diet on a regular pre-planned schedule
- taking a mental time-out to enjoy the moment

- taking deep, rhythmic breaths
- engaging in aromatherapy using pleasing scents and fragrances
- receiving a back rub or touch from a loved one
- thinking happy, positive thoughts
- following a lite approach to life
- spending time in a park or even just staring at trees

Getting Outside

Research shows that people are spending significantly less time outside. We are outside in a natural setting 25 percent less compared with just 20 years ago, with many negative consequences. Our overall sense of well-being is affected, because not only does nature reduce our feelings of being stressed, it has a host of positive effects on our body and mind. Including [5]:

- being happier
- being more creative
- feeling less depression
- feeling more connected, a greater sense of belonging
- having higher feelings of self-esteem
- feeling tranquility and calmness

Being in a natural setting is a great way to reduce your stress and improve your well-being. Just do it! It makes you feel better in so many ways.

Becoming More Self-Aware

Another great tool is to practice a high level of self-awareness, allowing you to momentarily detach yourself from the stress event and mitigate its effects before they are manifested in your body.[6] You can Take 5 and ask yourself, "Is this really so bad?" "What's the worst thing that could happen because of this?" Or tell yourself, "This too will pass." All of these statements are designed to take the edge off the stressor and allow it to dissipate or weaken before it can damage your brain or your body.

I used to experience an ongoing low level of chronic free-floating stress, not acute, just always there below the surface. This stress affected my ability to readily feel joy and happiness. What's more, it drove me to snack to try and counter its effects. This ongoing stress was exacerbated by an extremely high coronary calcium test score I received a few years ago. Rationally, I knew that the implications of a high test score were uncertain, and my doctor told me that my chance of having a heart attack were still quite low. Yet, these thoughts hid in the recesses of my mind and caused me unnecessary worry. The worry was unnecessary because I had never experienced even one symptom of heart distress and my diet lifestyle and exercise routines were already exactly what were prescribed to maintain an optimally heart-healthy life. Yet, this fear continued to persist and affect my life.

I needed a means to counter this stress and reduce the irrational worry that was discomforting and driving me to snack inappropriately. My solution was to proactively take, two Take 5 pauses at mid-day and early evening for the avowed purpose of reducing my stress and alleviating my worry. It worked and still does. The rhythmic deep in and out breathing, while silently reciting my "Peace Now" mantra, takes the edge off of my stress and relaxes my bodymind. During my 5-minute pause, I further reflect on the fact that my real coronary risks are low and that my diet and exercise practices are already extremely heart-healthy. To further combat this, beyond my regular twice a day Take 5 pauses, if I become aware of feeling stress induced anxiety about my heart health, I stop right then and there and Take 5. This always works to blunt the effects of my worry.

Stress in the Workplace

Stress in your workplace is pervasive. It is generated by several factors that mutually reinforce their effect to create a stressful work environment. The stress you face at work comes from:

- unrealistic deadlines
- involvement in the drama of office politics
- tiring over the course of the day
- a lost sense of personal control
- aggravations initiated by a dysfunctional manager
- unresolved issues and concerns in our personal lives

Small amounts of stress at work can be positive, prompting you to get accomplished, but, when it accumulates day in and day out, it can:

- wear you out
- diminish creativity and productivity
- make you irritable

- deplete your mental energy and willpower.

Feeling stressed also makes you much more likely to succumb to the temptation to snack.

How can you counter these stress-induced snack-attack cravings in the workplace? It starts with reducing the accumulation of stress you experience so you can keep your willpower and resolve at a satisfactory and effective level.

Take 5 to Break Your Stress
There is another innovative activity you can engage in to mitigate the effects of stress, especially in the workplace (although it will work at home equally well). I call it a Take 5 break.

Here is where the five-minute Take 5 break can be so useful. The purpose is to utilize a very brief self-intervention, periodically throughout your workday. You should use this technique at least once in the morning and once in the afternoon. To maximize its effect, however, use it every two hours during your workday.

Here is how it works. First, set up your workspace environment to facilitate the process as follows:

- lock your door (if you have one), or flip over a sign on your cubicle that says "Taking 5."
- turn off the lights if you can.
- mute your office telephone and your cell phone.
- lean back in your chair.
- set a timer for five minutes.
- close your eyes.

Now the stage is set for this mini-meditative exercise, as follows:

1. Take 60 seconds to progressively tense and release your body's muscles.
2. Take a deep breath in through your nose and silently repeat a mantra (a phrase) such as "peace" or "relax," hold the breath for about five seconds and as you exhale through your mouth, complete your mantra with the word "now."
3. Exhale completely, emptying your lungs of air.

4. Repeat steps 2 and 3 until the timer goes off.

This accomplishes several things. The Take 5 break:

- relaxes your body
- calms and unclutters your mind
- improves your focus
- generates mental energy that helps to replenish your willpower and self-control

By re-setting your brain, you feel a sense of rejuvenation that has a number of benefits. By managing and reducing your stress level, you boost and replenish your willpower, allowing you to rededicate yourself to whatever work task you were doing with increased energy and creativity. The Take 5 break has the potential to be a significant productivity booster.

In terms of the Whole Brain Diet Lifestyle, the Take 5 break defuses the emotional hunger you face when under stress. You greatly increase the odds that you can bypass the unhealthy snack more than if you had not taken this pre-emptive stress reducing step. Psychologically and physiologically, the Take 5 break is a brain-smart activity that benefits you during your workday (and is useful during non-workday times as well).

The Take 5 break is something you can do to reduce your workplace stress preemptively. But, when I was working, I encountered many instances where I instantaneously created my own stress by being an impatient and sometimes impulsive person. This impatience caused me distress by prompting me to engage in inappropriate and premature responses. Sometimes just by the thought and worry that I might do this, even when I was not actually doing so caused me stress. More times than I care to recall, I fired back an email, in response to a colleague's email to me that I dearly wished I had not. What's more, these were sometimes directed to colleagues whose friendship and support I needed and relied on.

If only I had known then, what I know now about using the Take 5 technique to defuse an emotionally-driven response in the heat of the moment, it would have saved me a lot of grief and aggravation. Take 5 is exactly the right tool to use to shift one's response mode from being unconscious and semi-automatic, to a conscious and deliberative state. This is a state where you have a real opportunity to make a better, more reasoned decision on how you want to proceed. The philosopher Viktor Frankl said that there is always a space between stimulus and response where you have a real choice on how to proceed. Take 5 makes this space very discrete and very real so you can always exercise this freedom of choice.

Other Stressors and Stress Effects

In the workplace, a highly time-consuming and often distracting task is the constant barrage of emails that cause you to stop what you are doing and attend to them. In her book *The Happiness Track*, Stanford University's Emma Seppala offers some thoughts on how to minimize this distraction and the resulting stress.[8] You might turn off the automatic notification that alerts you to an incoming email and access your email only once per hour, or even only a few times per day. Further, businesses should utilize priorities for emails that truly indicate when immediate attention is required, thus allowing all other emails to be attended to later on.

Merely having a smartphone in your presence, whether you look at it or not, is distracting and may add to your stress level. If you are not actually using your phone, mute it, place it in a drawer, away from your line of sight.

Stress creates a heaviness of mind and being, the antithesis of liteness and weightlessness. Controlling, managing and reducing the stress you experience is a very brain-smart thing to, helps to sustain a lite approach to life and is a powerful aid to maintain and build your mental energy, willpower and self-control.

The Mid-Afternoon Slump

Using the Take 5 break to defuse your stress is important and highly beneficial, but there are other times during the workday that also need to be addressed. All employees take breaks during which they have social conversations with fellow employees, which is a pleasant and stress-reducing activity. I recommend that you coordinate your break time with your work friends to minimize the disruptions it may cause. In fact, it would be even better if corporate management provided a social break time that all employees were encouraged to take, and most would take if approved. This break time would logically be during the mid-afternoon to correspond to the natural ebb and flow of our circadian biorhythms that tend to slump at this time of day. This is when employees' mental energy naturally drops off dramatically and they become more easily distracted, with a consequent falling off in productivity and creativity.

A formally sanctioned mid-afternoon break would work on many levels for both the employer and the employee. The employer gains employees whose brains and spirits are re-energized, resulting in better late-day morale and subsequently better productivity. The employees get to do what they often do anyway (i.e., socialize), but may feel guilty about doing. At the same time, they can "fill their plate" with a helping of social connectivity, instead of falling prey to unhealthful snacks.

This simple policy would turn a natural, negative, low productivity period into a huge win-win scenario for both management and their workers. Radical, yes, but an idea backed by both science and common sense.

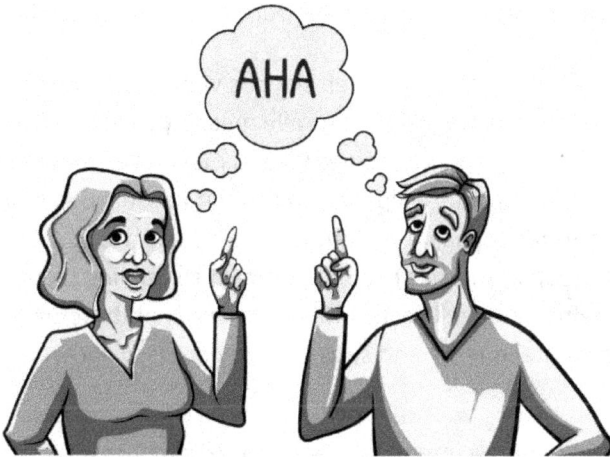

- Stress has negative physiologic effects only when your brain actually perceives the event as stressful. You can use your self-awareness to practice what I call the STOP technique. Namely, to stop from feeling the stress: Stop, Think, Observe, Process it, then detach from it and let it float away. The more you practice this technique, the more automatic and useful it becomes.
- Stress is a powerful force that reduces your mental energy and depletes your willpower and resolve to stand strong against a high-sugar, high-calorie snack-attack. Stress is pervasive and insidious, but you can learn how to minimize and manage it.

Chapter 15: Sleep
Sleep is <u>not</u> your enemy; <u>sleep is your ally.</u>

Sleep: An Often Overlooked Factor
A completely independent factor often overlooked when trying to effect a significant change in your lifestyle is the role and impact of sleep.[1] Most adults need seven to eight hours of sleep per night. When your sleep regularly falls below six hours, hormonal changes may take place in your body. There are two hunger-related hormones whose levels are affected: ghrelin and leptin.[2]

- Ghrelin stimulates your appetite, and when you regularly do not get enough sleep its level in your body is increased.
- Leptin levels tend to fall when your sleep level is not adequate; it tends to act as a hunger inhibitor.

Another key reason getting enough sleep is vital to enjoying a healthy lifestyle is that adequate sleep generally means you are well-rested. When you are well-rested, your willpower level is maximized and at its peak.[3] Being tired depletes your willpower, making it harder to eat well, eat sensibly and to resist the many temptations to eat badly. Avoiding poor and inadequate sleep is another highly important sustaining tactic. But more than that, being very well-rested via good sleep habits actually helps to build one's mental energy and subsequently one's willpower and self-control.

Being well-rested is an important regulator of alertness, boosting your mood and promoting a liteness in spirit. Not getting enough sleep promotes weight gain. Of course, if you are up in the middle of the night, you are also increasing your accessibility to food and snacking when your willpower is greatly diminished. Snacking at this time tends to be more unhealthy and higher simple-carb/sugar and calorie laden than at other snacking occasions.

Sleep and Cardiovascular Conditions
A large study of the Dutch population found a very high correlation between getting an adequate amount of sleep (7-9 hours per night) and fewer incidences of cardiovascular conditions.

The most impressive reduction in negative events was found among those who both followed a healthy lifestyle (defined as a healthy diet, exercise, not smoking and moderate alcohol consumption) and got adequate sleep. Among this group, cardiovascular events were reduced by 65 percent and fatal cardio-events by an astounding 83 percent, compared with those who did not follow a healthy lifestyle (including getting adequate sleep).

Truly impressive, however, is that among the segment who got adequate sleep, but did not otherwise follow all of the other healthy lifestyle factors, cardio events were still very significantly reduced. Good sleepers still experienced a level of protection equal to more than half of that experienced by those who followed all five healthy lifestyle activities.

Additionally, not getting adequate sleep has other negative effects, including[5]:

- Making you more irritable and more likely to be depressed
- Boosts likelihood of chronic illness resulting in increased probability of premature death
- Exacerbates the effects of feeling hangry

Sleep and Your Genes
Not getting enough sleep can alter the expression of your genes. In fact, getting enough sleep has been identified as a lifestyle behavior that helps to deter or delay the onset of Alzheimer's disease. Sleep is that important! Getting enough sleep optimizes the hormones that affect your appetite. It also is very friendly and protective to your heart as well as your brain.

Insomnia versus an Interrupted Sleep Pattern-They Are Not the Same
It is widely reported that many people experience insomnia, an inability to fall to sleep quickly, and/or waking up prematurely and not being able to get back to sleep.

Our pre-historic ancestors did not sleep through the night in one uninterrupted pattern.[6] Some experts who study these early humans suggest that they fell asleep after the sun went down and the sky darkened; woke up after four to five hours, engaged in some activity for an hour or two and then went back to sleep until sunrise. This behavioral imprint is still present in our brains today. That is why for many people the greater issue is falling back to sleep after awakening, rather than the ability to fall asleep in an acceptable time period. Enjoying eight-plus hours of uninterrupted sleep is largely a myth for many of us. The sleep-promoting tips below help you to fall off to sleep more quickly and sleep more soundly.

First, be sure your bedroom environment is optimized to promote sleep. For example, be sure that your bedroom:

- Is dark. Light interferes with sleep, and this includes clock numerals, computer screens, phones and all other lighted electronic devices. Shut them down all a minimum of a half-hour before bed.
- Is kept cool. Research indicates that a temperature around 60 to 65 degrees Fahrenheit may be optimal for most people.
- Remains quiet. If neighborhood noise regularly intrudes, consider a white noise machine that can mask many annoying sounds.
- Has a very comfortable bed and pillow. Sleep is too important, and a good quality bed or pillow is worth the investment.
- Has a bed used only for sleep and sexual relations. Non-sleep activity like watching television or reading gives your brain misleading signals. Your brain loves consistency and routine, so when it comes to sleep, be sure to give it what it needs.

Second, Take 5 to make a to-do list for the next day to minimize the likelihood that intrusive and worrisome thoughts hinder your falling asleep or falling back to sleep if you awake. There is nothing worse than tossing and turning, ruminating on everything you need to remember to do the following day.

Third, if you are prone to worry and fret about current or future events, write them down and literally put them into a box and close the lid. Metaphorically, this puts them aside to worry about some other time, not when you are trying to fall asleep. Worry is productive only if it spurs you to take an action you might otherwise not take. When you are trying to go to sleep, worry can only disrupt getting to sleep quickly and staying asleep longer.

When you enter your bed to sleep follow the same relaxation protocols as utilized in the Take 5 break. This may sound simple, but it has profound effects. The process calms and relaxes your body and brain and keep unwanted and potentially intrusive thoughts out of your mind. This mini-meditative practice works to combat insomnia, especially if you use it regularly and train your brain to respond by allowing you to fall asleep more quickly or fall back to sleep more easily if you awaken.

To fall asleep more rapidly establish a bedtime routine that your brain comes to expect and associates with your intent to fall and stay asleep. Routine and consistency make your brain happy, and a happy brain can help promote a restful night's sleep.

If you are a person of a certain age (you know who you are) who typically gets up once or twice a night to use the bathroom, a couple of other tips may help. First, always use a very low-brightness night light in your bathroom. A bright light may falsely alert your brain that morning is coming, and it is time to rise. On your way to the bathroom and until you return to your bed, repeat your favorite mantra, such as the word "peace." This helps to occupy your brain so that you do not dwell on unwanted thoughts that might pop into your head and prevent your falling back to sleep.

Waking up in the middle of the night can be frustrating when you can't fall back asleep and tossing and turning. One night in the midst of just such a circumstance, after endlessly staring at a darkened ceiling, I had a revelation that not only could I use Take 5 to facilitate my initially falling asleep, I could use it again to help me return to sleep. I tried it and it worked. Five minutes of deep in and out breathing, accompanied by repeating a mantra like "Peace Now," crowded out and blocked other potential random thoughts from entering my consciousness and demanding my attention. Breathing deeply and repeating this mantra works to clear my mind, calm my body and soothe my spirit, allowing me to re-enter a blissful state of slumber. While this does not work every time, it does work often. Take 5 is a great tool to quiet an unquiet mind long enough for me to fall back to sleep and it can do the same for you as well.

A friend of mine once said, "sleep is your ally." Getting enough sleep is certainly an ally to making and sustaining transformational changes to your lifestyle.

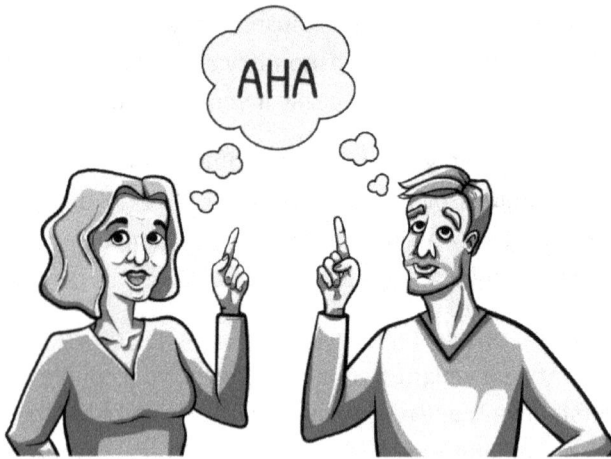

- Few things have the power of sleep to both increase mental energy and willpower when you are well-rested and to deplete it when you are tired. Sleep is critical to your weight loss, your health and your overall sense of well-being. Science does not totally understand sleep, but its critical importance to our health is undeniable.
- Give your brain the 7-8 hours of sleep per night that it craves and needs, and it rewards you daily by rejuvenating the mental and physical energy that carries you through your day.

Chapter 16: Compassion

Compassion directed inward is self-love, and this makes your brain very happy.

What Is Compassion?

A feeling that you can use to reinforce and translate your positive intentions into action is the greatly under-appreciated power of compassion. Compassion is the love, care and attention we typically think of as being created for and directed toward others, or from them to you. But you can also direct a compassionate intent toward yourself. It is a manifestation of self-respect and self-love. Mother Teresa was quoted as saying, "Never worry about numbers. Help one person at a time and always start with the person nearest you."[1] I choose to interpret this to mean always start with yourself. Importantly, self-compassion can be valuable in encouraging you to follow through on your intentions to change your behavior and your lifestyle.

Compassion can be created in unbounded quantities, and, serendipitously, the more often you create a compassionate intent for yourself or others, the easier it becomes to do it again. As the Beatles said, "The love you take is equal to the love you make."[2] Much has been written about the power of compassion. As comedienne Lucille Ball once said, "Love yourself first and everything else falls into line."[3]

Benefits of Expressing Compassion

Some of the positive benefits of creating compassion for yourself or directed to others is that compassion has real physical, emotional and spiritual benefits for both those who create it and for those who receive it.

These benefits include:

- Better physical health
- A sense of improved well-being
- A lift to the spirit and mood
- An increased desire to care for one's self
- Increased willpower and resolve
- Reducing the level of stress you experience
- Increasing one's personal happiness
- A positive spillover effect enhancing one's relationships

- An increase in longevity[4]

Creating compassion for yourself naturally correlates with an increased desire and will to take better care of yourself, and this aids you in realizing your goal of adopting a healthier Whole Brain Diet Lifestyle. Your willpower and resolve are magnified, and your ability to stay the course and persevere until your new positive behaviors take root are enhanced. Creating compassion and directing it inward toward yourself is another powerful maximizing step to boost your mental energy and to build and sustain your willpower and self-control.

You can even use Take 5 to facilitate directing compassionate thoughts inward to yourself. An excellent time to direct some love and attention to yourself is during a self-imposed five-minute Take 5 pause. Having positive thoughts about yourself feels good and boosts your inclination to take better care of yourself.

The old adage says that it is better to give than to receive. But when you create compassion and direct it inward toward yourself, you can actually both give and receive at the same time. Compassion directed inward helps to infuse your subconscious and align it with your conscious, deliberate intent, building an unstoppable force that propels you forward in your quest to effect behavioral change(s) in your life.

Compassion directed inward feels good, boosts your self-esteem, raises your mood and facilitates adopting a lite lifestyle, as these mental states are emblematic of being positive and lite in your orientation toward life. It also creates a positive feedback loop in which expressing self-compassion encourages you to adopt a lite lifestyle, which feeds back into boosting your self-compassionate feelings.

How Does Self-Compassion Work to Better Your Life?
Adam Grant in his book *Give and Take,* offers some insight into this process.[5] The central premise of his book is that givers who also maintain an active mind-set of self-interest tend to be the most successful in business and in life. When a person of their own free will creates compassion and lives a life of giving to others (and to themselves as well), their lives become better.

Grant postulates that giving, as in creating compassion for yourself, leads to greater personal happiness and gives meaning to your life, increasing your willpower and motivating you to work harder toward your goals. My take on this is that directing compassionate intent inward makes your brain happy. A happy brain releases neurotransmitters (like dopamine) that make you feel good and feel better. This leads to repeating the same behaviors that made the brain happy in the first place, and the self-reinforcing cycle continues.

Another highly positive act of self-compassion is to make it a habit to express gratitude on a daily basis. Emma Seppala, in her book *The Happiness Track*, explains how the act of being grateful is highly correlated with the feeling of positive emotions.[6] She states that gratitude is a source of strength and improves your well-being. These positive feelings act to boost your mental energy.

One day when I was especially down about something I cannot even recall, my wandering mind turned toward how much I actually had to be grateful for. Not just the fact that I had adequate food and safe shelter, but I also had great relationships with friends and a highly supportive family. Just reaffirming what I knew, but, took for granted, was a revelation that immediately made me feel better. My outlook improved and my mood was lifted. I was determined to not take for granted any longer those things, both small and large, that made my life better.

I sought a way to incorporate feelings of gratitude into my daily life and routine and I hit upon a solution. I resolved to employ Take 5 daily. It is the last thing I do after I get in bed. I reflect on all that I was grateful for and those whom I should thank for the graciousness and kindness they showed to me. It leaves me with good, positive feelings and a mental state primed for sleep.

Creating compassion and gratitude is very brain smart, take advantage of their natural power to help you change your life for the better.

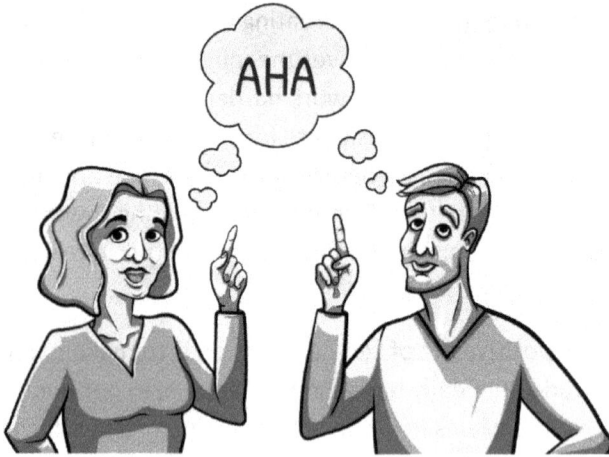

- Compassion at an individual level makes your life better; at a corporate level, it makes employees happier and more productive; and at a societal level it makes the world a better place to live. The power of compassion to improve your life is becoming more evident, although it is still very under-appreciated. Practice it daily and make realizing your dietary lifestyle transformation more likely.
- When you regularly practice compassion that you direct inward toward yourself, you are naturally more motivated to make healthier food choices to nourish your body and your spirit. Practicing self-compassion truly has no negative unintended consequences; it is always a winning proposition.

Chapter 17: Embodied Cognition and Lifestyle Change

Every aspect of your environment affects your feelings, thoughts and behavior, often in unexpected ways.

Free will is an illusion that we cling to because it makes us feel good to think that we are the master of our domain,[1] i.e., that we consciously make all of our own decisions and decide our own fate. The truth is that we are highly influenced by our emotions and the unconscious cues and triggers that precipitate our behaviors without active, deliberate thought. Much of what we say and do is influenced by the external and internal environment in which we live. It is a critical and little understood driver that shapes our daily life.

Most of us live our lives blissfully unaware of these influences. Even when you have some awareness and recognize them, you cannot completely eliminate their impact and remove all of their influence. But you do not have to be an unwitting pawn to these environmental influences; you can mediate their effects. You can, with effort, construct your environment to make it complement instead of obstructing your long-term objectives for lifestyle transformation.

First become aware of the power and influence of the environment over your decision making and behavior. Second, learn to use tools and tactics to consciously and actively mold your environment to further your long-term goals.

Not many people know much about embodied cognition, why it matters or how it can influence your life. One definition describes it as how the sensory experience of your environment influences your rational mind, thoughts and behavior.[2] There is an intimate interconnection among your senses, bodily states and cognition (that is, how and what you think). This can have profound effects on your attitudes, beliefs and subsequently your behavior. Sensory inputs including temperature, weight, texture, shape, smell, touch, color, sound, size and others affect your mental state and behavior. Sometimes the connection is obvious; other times the connection is more subtle and even counterintuitive.

Interestingly, metaphors can encode sensory stimuli and rapidly communicate sometimes complex ideas in an easily and widely understood fashion. When you want to distance yourself from a problem or incident you might say, "I wash my hands of the whole matter." Metaphorical expressions activate the same brain regions as the actual physical sensations of feeling washing your hands clean.[3] In this way, your sensory experiences affect how you think, what you believe and subsequently how you behave.

The principles and ideas associated with embodied cognition also have real and substantive effects on your eating behaviors, your tendency to overeat and even your likelihood of adopting a new, healthier diet lifestyle. You can consciously and deliberately employ these ideas in your daily life in a way that furthers your avowed intention to eat smart – eat in moderation.

Several ways to apply this include:

- Configuring your external and internal environment in a way that proactively uses the principles of embodied cognition.
- Using metaphorical statements associated with embodied cognition to reinforce your will and resolve to eat smart – eat in moderation.

Configuring Your External Environment
There are many elements of your external environment that influence how you feel and subsequently how you think and behave.

Eating Venue: Ambient Temperature and Lighting
The environment of the room you eat in influences your eating behavior. It's easy to understand that if your eating venue is too cold, you tend to eat quickly and likely too fast to reach a state of satiety. A warm room may be more beneficial than a cold room for two reasons. First, studies show that eating in warmer temperature leads to lower consumption. Second, the feeling of warmth tends to make you more open toward suggestion, more accepting and agreeable to following your own intentions, therefore repeating your Take 5 mantras in a warmer room is more effective.[4]

A brightly lit venue is preferable to one that is a dark. Psychologically, you are more likely to cheat in a dimly lit room and to linger over your meal a longer time. Dim lighting also promotes eating more of less healthy food offerings.[5] In bright light, you are less able to hide your gluttony from yourself and others. More light is also associated with a brighter mood and more positive feelings. When you have a choice, choose to eat in a room with a lot of light (especially natural light).

Chairs and Tables

The construction of your kitchen (or restaurant) tables and chairs also makes a difference. Whether or not the chair and table is hard and unyielding or soft and cushy makes a difference. A soft, cushy chair makes you feel more agreeable and more sociable and more likely to continue to eat as long as your companions are eating, while a harder surface makes you more stringent and less amenable to cheating and overeating. A hard chair and table act to unconsciously harden your resolve to eat smart – eat in moderation.[6] Of course, this can be taken too far. If your chair is super hard and extremely uncomfortable, you may tend to eat too quickly, prompting you to overeat.

Eating Utensils, Plates and Glasses

We already know, using heavier utensils, plates and glasses, gives food a more substantial feel, while smaller forks and spoons make you feel like you are consuming more. It is also true that we typically perceive food as higher quality and more palatable when we eat with newer and higher-quality utensils, plates and glasses. Buy a set of highly used tableware that looks and feels old to diminish your perceptions of food palatability and thereby dissuade you from overeating.[7] Additionally, the influence of color makes a difference in the portion size served and the amount you end up eating.[8] This is particularly true when you are a bit distracted and paying less attention to what you are doing.

Eating Room Color, Accessories and Floor Plan

The color of the room you are eating in and the accessories that adorn the walls influence your eating behavior. A soft, pastel blue is calming and just makes you feel good.[9] On the walls of your kitchen, place photos of natural scenes like woods, streams, mountains. These types of scenes are associated with uplifted spirits and the kind of good feelings that boost your mental energy and self-control, helping you to eat smart – eat in moderation.[10] Additionally, you can place a mirror strategically so you can see yourself eat. Seeing your image makes you less likely to cheat and overeat, as you are more mindful of what and how much you are eating.[11]

Your eating venue's floor plan may affect how much you eat and your ability to eat in moderation. A very open floor plan encourages greater food consumption, especially when additional, unserved food is still visible where you are eating. A highly open space makes you feel more expansive, less psychologically restricted and thus open to eating more. It is also a good idea to keep your unserved food separate from where you are eating – for example, keep the food in the kitchen while you are eating in your dining room.[12]

Listening to Music While Eating Your Meal

There are conflicting views on listening to music during your meal. On the one hand, you do not want to be distracted, because you want to be mindful to savor and eat slowly. On the other hand, slow tempo that lasts for about a half an hour can pace your meal. The music can cue you to eat slowly and spread your eating out over the whole length of the musical piece. What you do not want to do is to listen to raucous, high-energy, high-tempo music that distracts your attention away from your eating and prompts you to eat too quickly.[13]

Configuring Your Internal Environment and Your Personal Space

There are many steps you can take after you understand how your internal environment and your personal space influences your decision making and behavior to use this awareness to your advantage. With this knowledge, you can take conscious and deliberate actions to make use of these influences, which in turn help you to more easily achieve your Whole Brain Diet Lifestyle goals.

Dampening the Visual and Olfactory Appeal of Food

It is no secret that our appetite is whetted by how our food looks and smells. Food that looks and smells good increases the food's perceived palatability, our feelings of eating enjoyment and may propel us to overeat. We do not want to take all of the pleasure out of eating good-tasting food. But if you can make it look less appetizing and aromatically alluring, you have a better chance to control your impulses to eat too quickly and overeat. You can wear sunglasses when you eat. Especially glasses with a dark grey or brown tint.

How Your Posture Affects Your Perceptions

The act of sitting tall and straight in your chair (i.e., not slumped down), gives you a greater sense of control and of efficacy and consequently a greater ability to eat as you intended and to eat in moderation.[14] In the realm of embodied cognition, even your posture can affect your perceptions and ultimately your behavior.

Harvard Business School professor Amy Cuddy, author of the book *Presence* and the promulgator of the theory behind Power Posing suggest you can take a Power Posing stance, while repeating a phrase such as, " ("Your Name") is in control of his/her eating. He/she has the power and the ability today, and every day, to eat smart – eat in moderation." The use of this expansive posturing increases your confidence in your ability to eat in moderation, as having a firm belief and expectation of being able to do something has a credible effect on your actual ability to do it.[16]

Pre-Meal Routine

Adding to your pre-meal routine, imagine that you are eating, savoring and enjoying the meal to take the edge off your hunger and allow you to reach satiety a little sooner. When you vividly imagine a behavior, the neurons in your brain are activated similarly to when you actually physically engage in the same behavior.[16]

Add to this routine to repeat statements that reinforce your intentions to eat in moderation, while you simultaneously squeeze on a hard ball. The sensation of hardness produces a metaphorical hardening of your resolve and intent, focusing your attention on following through on your desired objectives.[17]

Using Metaphorical Statements

You can also consciously employ metaphors and metaphorical statements to help reinforce your will and resolve to achieve your goal to eat smart – eat in moderation. Before meals, you can repeat metaphorical statements in terms of steeling yourself, hardening your convictions and toughening your resolve.

Examples of Useful Metaphorical Statements

- "(*Your Name*) is like a soldier in a war against his/her excess weight, against his/her obesity. He/she is engaged in a battle with his/her cravings that he/she can, will and must win."
- "(*Your Name*) has a steely resolve and an ironclad will to follow his/her lifestyle goals today and every day."
- "(*Your Name*) has the heart of a lion, Herculean strength and the will of a mother grizzly protecting her cubs and he/she chooses to eat smart —eat in moderation now and always."

These metaphors strengthen your intentions. They activate a psychological state in which your expectations in your beliefs are enhanced, and this enhancement makes carrying out your intentions more likely to happen.

Other Considerations

I encourage the rest of you not to ponder how and why embodied cognition works. Just implement the recommendations that you believe you can viably incorporate into your daily routine. There is some evidence that the effects of embodied cognition work on a deeply unconscious level and that your conscious beliefs do not interfere with your thoughts and behavior.

Some of the recommendations I have made will likely make eating somewhat less enjoyable, less fun. You may ask whether you really want to take away from one of life's greatest pleasures. You need to answer that question for yourself. But if you are seriously overweight and your weight is threatening your overall health, your self-image and your well-being, then the answer likely is, yes you do.

You can adopt just those tools and tactics that you feel make the most sense for you, which you can live with and incorporate into your life. As your weight comes down to a level that you can comfortably and healthfully live with, you can also choose to selectively eliminate some tactics you might find burdensome and see how that works for you. The Whole Brain Diet Lifestyle is intended to be a lifelong journey, but it can evolve to meet your needs over time. It is not intended to imprison you, to handcuff you with a rigid set of inflexible rules.

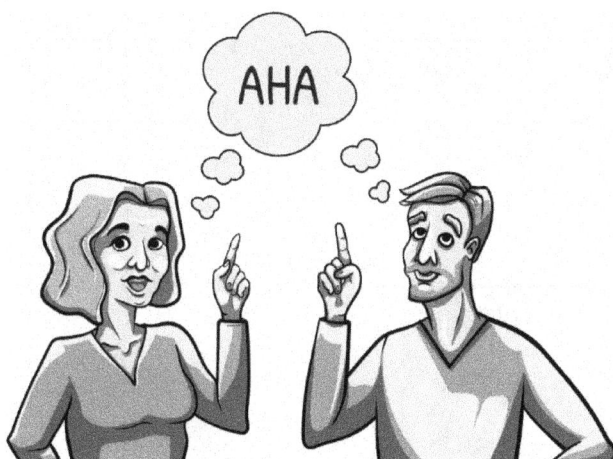

- Some of the tactics and principles of cognitive embodiment are counter-intuitive. Don't ponder them too deeply; just give them a try.
- There is no need to incorporate all of the tools and tactics in this chapter, just select those that seem most doable to you and the ones you feel you can employ for the long-run.

Part 4:

Additional Perspectives on the Whole Brain Diet Lifestyle

Chapter 18: Whole Brain Diet Lifestyle, Take 5 and Parents

Parents have a brief window of optimal opportunity to imprint positive dietary habits onto their children. Either use it or lose it, the choice is yours.

This is not intended as a chapter about how to parent your child, but, what you can do as a parent on your child's behalf to affect their health and diet for the long-run. The seriousness of weight concerns among children is large and growing. More than 17 percent of kids and teens are considered obese and in total, 33 percent are overweight.[1] When you consider that calories from snacks alone have increased by over 400 calories a day between 1977 to 2006, it is hardly surprising.[2] An overweight or obese child is very likely to evolve into an overweight or obese adult.

Birth to Kindergarten: Unparalleled Opportunity

Parents have a unique, unparalleled opportunity in a narrow window of time, to influence their child's life. From before birth until perhaps kindergarten is a period during which parents, through their conscious, deliberate and planned interventions, can change their child's life forever. Before your child becomes socialized and imprinted with the values, preferences and behaviors of others, apply your own imprints to influence your offspring for life.

Your child is not born with a clean mental slate, as all of the instincts and drives of humans' long evolutionary history are already present. Choose to have a plan for your child before resistance and competition from conflicting or alternative viewpoints emerge. I maintain that you not only have the right to engage in this activity, but have the responsibility to do so.

The values, beliefs, attitudes and learning imparted to your children in their early years, have a unique advantage to be imprinted and internalized in a fashion that can last and affect for life. If you do not choose to exert this influence in a careful, planned approach, you influence your children anyway, but perhaps in ways you never intended nor can imagine.

Introduce you children to Take 5 when they reach kindergarten. At first, you can simply tell them to Take 5 and impose a five-minute pause before yielding to their snack demands. Later, you can simply remind them to Take

5 and praise their decision to do so. Finally, after continued reinforcement and usage, Take 5 becomes natural to them, and they may continue to employ it on their own.

Impact of Epigenetics on Your Child Prior to Conception

Livescience.com defines epigenetics as literally meaning, "on top of genetics. It refers to external modifications to DNA that turn genes 'on' or 'off.' These genes do not affect the gene sequence, but instead affect how cells 'read' genes."[3] What this means is that it may be possible to pass down these changes to future generations, if the changes occur in the sperm or egg cells. Most, but not all, epigenetic changes that occur in sperm and egg cells get erased when the two combine to form a fertilized egg, in a process called reprogramming. This reprogramming allows the cells of the fetus to start from scratch and make their own epigenetic changes. Scientists think some of the epigenetic changes in parents' sperm and egg cells may avoid the reprogramming process, and make it through to the next generation. This means that the food a person eats before they conceive may affect their future child.[4]

Although the field is new and unfolding, it is becoming increasingly apparent that parents, through the diet they consume prior to impregnation and gestation (and via other lifestyle choices as well), can affect the expression of genes in their unborn child. A diet very high in vegetables, fruits and complex carbs and low in processed sugar and other pre-sweetened foods may affect your child's preferences for certain foods after birth. This diet is not only more nutritious and sensible than one high in sugars and other junk foods, so why not follow it more rigorously prior to and during pregnancy?

A new, exciting study reported at a meeting of the APS (American Psychological Society), based on mouse research but thought to be applicable to humans, suggests that a pregnant women's exercise regimen could significantly affect the health of their unborn child. Specifically, regular exercise may give the unborn child a resistance to stress effects and improved insulin sensitivity with a material effect on their overall health. In a statement to the APS, the primary research investigator wrote, "Our findings highlight pregnancy as a sensitive period when positive lifestyle interventions could have significant and long-lasting beneficial effects on offspring metabolism and disease risk."[5]

Impact of Mother's Pre-birth Diet on Child's Life-long Food Preferences

Emergent research strongly suggests that a mother's diet while pregnant may have a significant and lasting impact on her baby's life-long food preferences. This research indicates that a mother whose diet is nutrient rich, varied and otherwise considered healthful transfers to her unborn child a preference and even an emotional connection with the same types of food. On the other hand, mothers whose diet is nutrient poor and loaded with high-simple-carb, high-sugar foods have a very different effect.

Pregnant women who consume an unhealthy diet may desensitize their child to the same tastes after they are born. These children, who are already endowed with an innate preference for sugar, need much higher quantities of these foods to derive the same level of pleasure from their consumption. This obviously is a contributing factor to childhood (and subsequently adult) overeating and obesity.

It is a provocative and compelling idea that mothers can significantly influence their child's food preferences while their child is still in the womb. Because of the evolutionary advantages to pre-historic survival, desire for sugar is hard-wired in the brain. As parents we can further magnify this preference and make it even harder to resist in our child's future, or we have a chance to reduce this preference by the action and behavior of the mother during pregnancy.

Research conducted at Yale University indicates that mothers who eat a high-fat diet during pregnancy affect the metabolism of their child after birth. The result of this unhealthy diet during pregnancy is a higher risk of lifelong obesity in their child. The mechanism of action may not be clear, but the result seems to support the premise that a mother's diet can have an enduring impact on the health and likelihood of obesity in their children.[6]

Children of women who breastfeed enjoy a more diverse array of flavors through the milk than those fed only by the bottle. This early exposure may confer on the baby a greater openness to accept a wider variety of tastes and flavors as children.

Children's Natural Preference for Sugar

The preference and craving for sugar are instinctive drives that is part of our DNA. Parents should not try to quash or eliminate this natural preference. But your do not have to reinforce and magnify your children's pre-existing sweet tooth. Do not engage in behaviors that cause your children to associate sweetness and sugar with reward.

Parents, whether deliberate or accidental, play a highly significant role in shaping children's lifelong diet lifestyle.[7] You, as parents, can position sweets as items that are consumed only on special occasions. They might still be coveted, but eaten only sparingly.

As Rudy Tanzi and Deepak Chopra postulate in their book *Super Brain*, automatic imprints are fashioned in our childhood and have an advantage as they become subconscious. With years of reinforcement, these thoughts and feelings often become part of a person's core self-image.[8] This imprinting can be positive, healthy and good for our children, or it can be negative, unhealthy and bad for them. Either way, childhood imprinting has a powerful effect on our children's behavior as teens and adults. Parents should have a deliberate approach to how this imprinting unfolds, and not leave it totally to chance.

How Parents Reinforce Their Children's Natural Craving

Sometimes, the reinforcement process starts immediately after birth. It doesn't take long for a mother of a reluctant milk or formula drinker to realize that sweetening the nipple (of the breast or bottle) with a little sugar stimulates the infant to suck harder and suck longer.

When the infant progresses to solid foods, the reinforcement often continues. Most infants show a natural preference for, and eat more completely and readily, strained fruits over strained vegetables. Naturally, a mother wants her child to eat as much as is prescribed, so she may serve her child the sweet food items over the vegetables.

As the child ages, the reinforcement process not only continues, but it often escalates and intensifies. Many children are notoriously poor eaters and either refuse to eat, or eat only a very limited quantity of food they do not naturally like. For them, this may include many slightly bitter and non-sweet vegetables and other non-sweetened food items. How often have you heard a mother try to reason with her children by offering them dessert if they eat what is on their plate and no dessert if they don't? Of course, the most desirable desserts are the high-simple-carb, high-sugar, high-calorie kind. This stimulus (i.e., refusal to eat) and response (i.e., promise of dessert), simply reinforces the connection between reward and sugar.

The lesson, sometimes unstated and non-verbalized but made crystal clear, is that sweet, high-sugar foods are desirable and very rewarding. Of course, eating a meal is only one situation where parents bribe their children with a sweet treat as a reward, there are many other circumstances where this is used as well.

The pleasure-and-reward circuits in children's brains light-up in delight when they consume (or even just think about consuming) high-sugar foods.[9] The more often a child is given a sweet treat, the more they want to receive it in the future, and the mind-body connection between sugar and reward strengthens.

Parents may also employ operant conditioning to try and reinforce their children's acceptance and consumption of fruits and vegetables and dissuade them from demanding pre-sweetened foods and snacks. For example, when your child eats his/her fruits and veggies, reward him/her with a kiss, a smile, a touch, verbal praise and/or soothing baby babble. This helps reinforce the desired behavior of your child eating highly nutritious, healthy foods. For most children, the more often they are given the opportunity to eat fruits and vegetables, the more often they will eat them and the more they eat them, the more they tend to like them and accept them over time.

At the same time, your child is never too young learn that a traditional, high-simple-carb, high-sugar, high-calorie dessert is intended for, and appropriate for, only special occasions like the weekly family post-Sunday dinner treat, or a birthday event. They may not get the point at first, but over time they absorb the lesson that sugary desserts/snacks are for special occasions only. Start young and be consistent, and your child learns the lesson.

As a parent, you can also give your child fruits that are high in natural sweetness, such as raisins, figs, dates and bananas. The purpose is twofold. First, it helps to satisfy their innate sweet tooth and make it easier for you to resist offering your child a highly processed and pre-sweetened snacks.

174

Secondly, if your children become more accustomed to the natural sweetness of fruit, they may find the artificial sweetness of processed, sugary deserts, unnaturally sweet and develop more of a preference for fruit.

As they become older and learn about the dangers and concerns concerning consuming too much sugar and eating too many calories, this early training helps them adhere to a healthful diet.

Of course, a parent's own relationship to and consumption of sweet foods, snacks and desserts also makes a real impact on their children. Children have a keen perception for what they see their parents do, as opposed to simply what their parents say. If your children see you rewarding yourself and immensely enjoying a sugary treat, they will also value these items more highly than they would otherwise.

Your children provide another very important reason for altering and improving your own lifestyle. You can help to teach your children that sweets and other high-sugar foods are most appropriate as real special treat items. Nothing says special better than an event that is reserved for specific and very limited occasions for you and them.

The goal is not to try and totally deny your children's natural sweet tooth. Rather, the goal is to use your conscious intent to reposition your children's indulgence in high-sugar foods to a special treat status, and thereby significantly reduce how often they consume these foods.

Parents are crucial in another way. As adult we often mistake our own emotional pain and negative emotional feelings for hunger when all we really need is to show ourselves some self-love, attention and caring, i.e., show ourselves some compassion.[10] We unintentionally promote the same association in our children. Consider the following scenario.

If you have an infant who is unable to articulate his/her wants and needs, how do you behave when they cry out, fuss or exhibit discomfort? If your first response and assessment is that they must be hungry, you may be confusing their cry for attention, care and/or touch, which is their emotional hunger, for physical hunger.[11] This leads to several potential issues. First, this may lead you to overfeed them and promote excess weight gain in their early youth. In the long-run, you may unintentionally reinforce the connection between emotional hunger and trying to fulfill this non-physical hunger with food. This behavior may cause your children, as adults, to try and fulfill their own emotional needs first with food, rather than the love, attention and care that they really need to show themselves. There is absolutely no doubt that overweight or obese children are highly likely to become overweight or obese adults.

If parents accept this highly important assignment as role models and molders of their children's behavior, the cycle of lifelong over-consumption of sugary foods and beverages can be broken, or at least slowed down. Of course, you and your children will still love sugar and will enjoy it on occasion, just not as often as you otherwise would be likely to do. Further, it helps make your children, as adults, more self-aware and better able to accurately discriminate between feelings of emotional hunger and legitimate feelings of physical hunger.

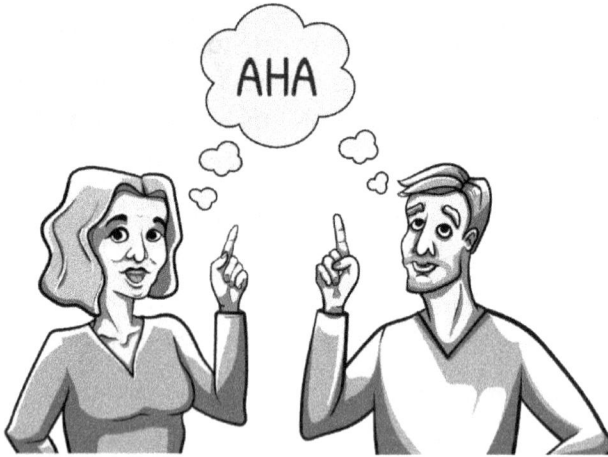

- Mothers and fathers are influencing their children's lives, sometimes permanently, by their own lifestyle choices prior to conception. Fat and highly stressed parents are more likely to produce heavy and stress-susceptible children. This should present you with one more compelling reason to transform your own dietary lifestyle, not just for yourself, but for the good of your unborn offspring as well.
- Very young children are like sponges. They hear your words, but they actually absorb and reflect your behaviors. When it comes to practicing a healthy diet lifestyle, you must not only talk the talk, but also walk the walk.

Chapter 19: Don't Drink a Calorie

Give up almost all sugary beverages (including soft drinks and juices) and exchange them for no-calorie beverages, such as water, tea or coffee.

High levels of sugar act on the brain's reward/pleasure receptors similar to a drug. Over time, sugar stimulates the brain to release less of the feel-good chemical neurotransmitter dopamine, requiring ever more of the same stimulator (i.e., sugar) to release the same quantity of this feel-good brain chemical in the future.[1] In this way, the brain learns to crave more sugar. Sugar in moderation is not an inherently bad thing, but too much can be toxic.

Sugar is ubiquitous in the American diet. There are over a dozen forms of sugar. This can take the form of simple table sugar, honey, molasses or corn syrup. The average Americans sugar consumption has been on a steady rise over the past few hundred years: in 1750 it was about four pounds per year; 1850, 20 pounds; 1994, 120 pounds; and today, around 156 pounds.[2] One teaspoon of sugar has 16 calories and one teaspoon of corn syrup has 19. In a 2,500-calorie daily diet, many nutritionists recommend that no more than 10 percent of total calories, or about 250 calories, come from any form of simple sugar. In the average adult diet today, we consume 42+ teaspoons per day, or 630 calories, translating to around 25 percent to 30 percent of our daily total calories.

Pounds of Sugar

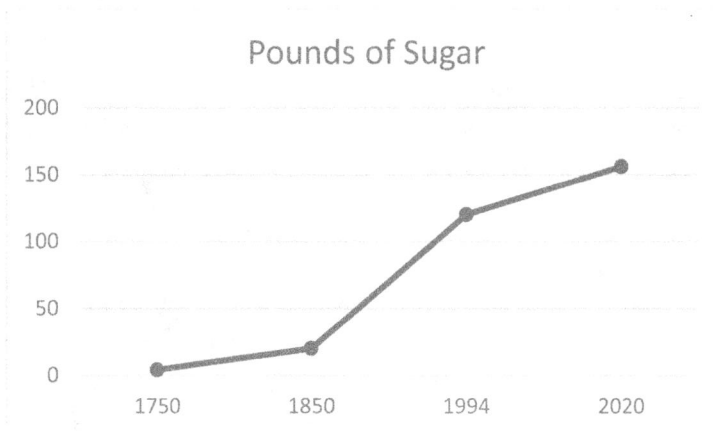

Why focus on sugary soft drinks? They have 10-11 teaspoons of added sugar, containing around 150 nutritionally empty calories per can. So, one can per day makes up 5 percent to 7 percent of a recommended daily calorie allotment, two cans about 10 percent to 14 percent. These calories do not have nutritional value, and excessive sugar consumption has many other negative consequences as well.

Sugar Can Be Toxic

In addition to the common culprits associated with excessive sugar intake like obesity and diabetes, too much sugar is associated with associated with some types of cancer (such as pancreatic and gallbladder) and heart disease as well.[3] Even worse, Harvard researchers attributed sugary drinks to 180,000 deaths a year worldwide, 25,000 in the United States alone.[4] Sugar is not only bad for your body, but deadly as well.

The mathematics of consuming a daily can of soda is highly dramatic and attention-getting. One can of 12-ounce soda or juice contains about 150 calories per 12-ounce serving. 150 calories per day, 365 days per year yields a grand total of 54,750 calories per year. At the conversion rate of 3,500 calories per pound, 54,750 extra calories per year translates into a theoretical annual gain of almost 16 pounds.

On paper, eliminating one can of sugary beverage per day causes you to avoid a potential gain of 16 pounds per year if you do not offset the calorie reduction by consuming more of other high-sugar, high-calories foods. This single change in your lifestyle reaps significant and enduring benefits to your weight and health, and by extension to your overall life and well-being.

While giving up your treasured soft drinks may not be easy, if you focus all of your attention, energy, willpower and resolve on this one behavior, you can do it. It could be life changing if you are a regular sugary beverage or juice drinker.

If you are unable or unwilling to adopt some of the many recommendations in this book, and you simply choose to give-up most sugary beverages, your life will be simplified and choices reduced. The certainty of knowing that you choose to not consume sugary beverages provides your brain with an assurance it likes. This makes your brain happy, and a happy brain is motivated to continue those behaviors that make it happy. Focusing on a single goal makes it more achievable.

It should also be noted that not all no-calorie beverages are created equal. Plain, unadulterated water is one of the best beverages. I personally dilute my water with a very small amount of juice to increase its palatability, but pure water (still or sparkling) is best. You might ask, how about, zero calorie, sugar-free diet soft drinks?

These may not be so benign for the body. A partial list of the negative consequences associated with consuming sugar-free diet drinks includes the following[5]:

- increased risk of type 2 diabetes
- increased craving for sugar, which leads to consuming more sugar in other foods, leading, paradoxically, to weight gain and obesity
- decreased kidney function
- possible damage at the cellular level
- decreased bone density
- a high acid level that erodes tooth enamel

Even more provocative are the research findings that sugar-free, diet soft drinks may not even be beneficial as a means of reducing calorie intake and losing weight. Purdue University researchers reviewed a total of 12 studies on diet soda. They found that diet soda, as is true of regular, sugary soda, is associated with type 2 diabetes, metabolic syndrome and heart disease. They also found evidence that diet soda does not even help the consumer lose weight. There is even some evidence that drinking diet soda cause weight gain.[6]

Why might this be true? Artificial sweeteners may trick the brain into believing it is receiving the real sugar the brain craves. When it does not get the real thing, it affects one's metabolism, increases craving for real sugar even more, and leads to over-consumption as a result.

The lesson here is that all soft drinks, whether sugar or sugar-free, have negative consequences and are bereft of positive nutritional value. It is best to avoid, or at least minimize their consumption. While 100 percent fruit juices are nutritionally superior to soft drinks, they still contain a lot of sugar, and their use should also be carefully monitored and controlled or eliminated.

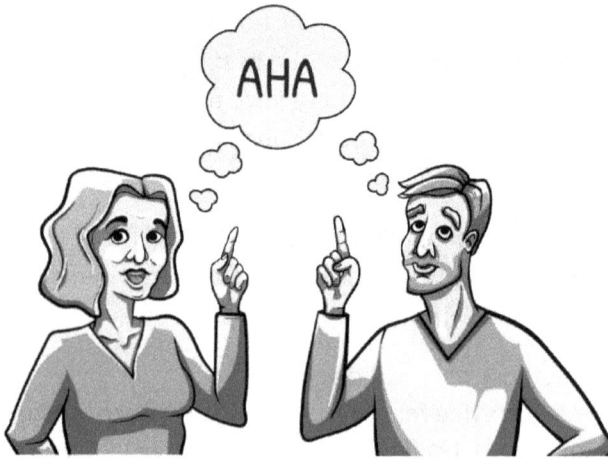

- Giving up all sugary beverages, soda and juice, is a brain-smart and nutritionally-smart choice.
- Diet soda may not only have no value as a weight loss aid, some evidence even suggests it may contribute to weight gain.

Chapter 20: The Thermostatic Weight Control Approach

Your brain loves certainty and routine. Give it what it wants by always having a dietary contingency plan in place.

The thermostatic approach to weight loss maintenance is a system I devised to maintain my weight once I've reached my goal. It involves the following facets.

It is critical that you weigh yourself regularly.[1] I weigh myself every morning, after undressing, before bathing and after using the bathroom. While this may seem extreme, regularly weighing yourself is key.

I also recommend that you keep a weight record journal. Just as many weight loss counselors recommend keeping a daily food journal of what you eat, keeping a daily record of your weight level is very useful. You will be able to discern your normal weight fluctuations, as well as having an undeniable signal of when your weight is moving beyond a typical fluctuating level. Nothing is more beneficial as a boost to your self-awareness and motivation, than being alert to a measurable weight gain while it is still small and more manageable.

There is another great tactic that may be more effective than simply seeing your weight as a number on a scale. It is the "skinny jeans" test, and it can be used both as a strong motivator to continue on your journey to a better, healthier lifestyle and as a concrete measure of how you are succeeding if weight loss is one of your goals. Buy a pair of jeans one size below your current size and try them one once or twice each month. When they start to feel more comfortable, it acts both to help you persevere in your quest and as an undeniable indicator of how well you are succeeding (or not). When these jeans feel comfortable start wearing them, buy the next smaller size and repeat the process.

This thermostatic approach is based on a few simple premises.

- You must be aware that you have gained an unacceptable amount of weight before you have an intent to lose it.
- Weight loss is more likely when you believe it can happen.

- A small weight loss is easier to imagine and truly easier to achieve than a larger weight loss.

The origination of the idea for my Thermostatic Theory of Weight Control evolved when I was walking through the living room of my home one very cold winter morning. Suddenly, the furnace kicked on and for the next 15 minutes the heat poured out. About a half hour later, the same cycle repeated itself as the outside air temperature was dropping. The thermostat turned on to activate the furnace in order to try and maintain the indoor temp at a steady level near the set point. I thought about the mechanical process whereby the smaller the temperature variance the thermostat is set for to activate, the more the furnace cycles on and off, but the easier it is to maintain a steady level indoor temperature.

Then, in a true "AHA Moment" I realized that the exact same logic could be applied to controlling and maintaining my weight. Simply, set a weight gain amount to act as an automatic trigger to initiate countervailing behaviors, via reducing caloric intake and/or increasing physical activity. Doing this helps you lose the weight gained and return to the set point you desire.

You may say that this is all obvious and hardly a breakthrough idea, but, what seems obvious after it is revealed, is not always so obvious beforehand. For me, this was a new thought. I have followed the principle of using this thermostatic approach ever since and it has helped me to maintain my weight in a fairly narrow range. When I do deviate from my set point, returning to my desired weight level is not difficult, as the variance is always small and not too hard to rectify.

Based on these truths, the thermostatic approach simply calls for setting a weight gain point where action and/or reaction is automatically activated. You lay down for yourself an inviolable rule, such as: You will never let yourself gain more than X pounds (e.g., three or four) before you engage in remedial action to lose that excess weight.

Of course, it is easier to state it than it is to implement it. But is a very sensible framework and attitude toward weight control. After you are able to transform your lifestyle and realize a weight you are happy with, this approach can greatly help you to maintain that weight level.

The Mental Game in Weight Control

Your brain controls your life and your behavior. You can use your brain to reinforce your intention to achieve a healthy weight and a fit body. Using principles of positive psychology and operant conditioning (i.e. setting up cues that trigger your behavior over time), can help you. It is best to construct your environment and life in a manner that encourages and promotes the behaviors you want to adopt.

Plan B

Everyone should have a Plan B that provides rules and options when you know you will be in situations where consuming excess food and calories is likely. These are situations where you probably expect to gain some weight or do not wish to deprive yourself or possibly put yourself in a socially awkward position. For example, going to a party, eating out in a restaurant, or being on vacation. Some of these may cause a short-term weight gain and others (like a vacation) can lead to experiencing a significant, long-term weight gain. This is where Plan B comes into play. Having a Plan B provides an easy and effective means to bring your weight back down after you have reached the upper limit of your range.

For every situation, where you expect to overeat and consume too much, you need a contingency plan. When you experience situation X, it automatically activates contingency activity Y. For example, if you will be in a situation that day where overeating is likely, you can do the following. Consciously force yourself to eat fewer high-calorie foods before your high consumption event. Don't skip a meal as this may propel you into a feeding frenzy later in the day.

At the same time, to complement your calorie reducing efforts, you can also increase your level of physical activity. Some combination of increased exercise and fewer calories can counter a bad eating occasion later in the day. Also, taking a walk after a meal not only aids your digestion, it distracts you from seeking a dessert.

A more serious eating challenge, like an extended vacation, calls for a more serious response and plan. Before I go on a vacation, where I know it is virtually impossible to resist the ample and very delicious food, I actively moderate what I eat a few weeks ahead. At the same time, I engage in activities that boost my metabolism to burn more calories. This way, I still enjoy myself while away without gaining a significant amount of weight that is hard to subsequently lose.

Another good addition to this plan is to make sure you exercise while you are on vacation. When I go on a cruise, I make sure to walk the promenade deck that circles the ship multiple times per day and to utilize the gym.

Fat Sunday into Skinny Monday

You might have heard of Fat Tuesday, but I want to introduce is the notion of a Fat Sunday into a Skinny Monday. On any given day (be it a Sunday or any day of the week), when you over-indulge, overeat and/or binge, the next day or two should be a day of deliberate, compensating behavior. Specifically, you should strive to limit the damage by eating fewer than normal calories over the next couple of days and moderately increasing your level of physical activity or exercise. The goal is not to completely offset the previous splurge in calories. The goal is to limit the additional calories.

Do not use this technique as a rationalization to over-indulge. But never overeating is not realistic. When it does occur, it makes sense to automatically engage in a countervailing behavior. You might still gain some weight, but it will be less. Also, the weight you gain comes off easier as the amount gained is less burdensome to lose.

These contingency plans simplify your life and reduce decision-making complexity, thereby helping to sustain your mental energy, willpower and self-control. The certainty of having pre-planned your behavioral responses to various challenging situations is an excellent, sustaining strategy to minimize depletion of your mental energy and willpower.

Daily Psychological Reinforcing Activities

Following a daily ritual of psychological reinforcement using scientifically validated principles can also be very beneficial.[2] This includes following a daily routine that you should try to do every night pre-bed and every morning post-awakening.

Pre-bed and post-awakening ritual

You should repeat out loud or silently to yourself, a series of statements that reinforce your commitment and positive intention to follow a healthy and sensible long-run Whole Brain Diet Lifestyle. These statements should include some of the following:[3]

- (*Your Name*) Takes 5 every time he/she feels a craving to eat high-sugar, high-calorie foods.
- (*Your Name*) rejects his/her *Fat* brain and chooses to follow the dictates of his/her *Skinny* brain!

You can also benefit from viewing images of people who look healthy and well.[4] One highly effective technique is to look at an old photo of yourself. While you can never reverse the aging process, you can aspire to be as vital and healthy as you were when you were younger. This helps you to follow and adhere to your contingency plans when needed.

Use of Rewards and Penalties

Similar to the reward system built into the weight loss phase of your Whole Brain Diet Lifestyle, a reward/penalty system can be applied to weight maintenance.

After you have reached a weight level that you consider to be good and healthy for your body and brain, you may give yourself (and/or a significant other) a reward/penalty for staying within this range over the next month, six months, year, and so forth. The longer you are able to maintain your ideal weight range, the bigger the reward you give to yourself.

Use both rewards and penalties. Research shows that your brain and pleasure circuits respond favorably to a positive incentive, such as a reward, but strives even more to avoid a punishment, such as a penalty for bad behavior.[5] There is no reason that you cannot continue to use this reward/penalty approach throughout your lifetime.

What If You Slip and Have a Relapse?

It is important to accept that we are all human with all the frailties and foibles that come with this territory. To fall off the healthy food consumption bandwagon is very human, and we will all likely do so sometimes. The key is to not beat yourself up too much. If you do, you are more likely to throw in the towel, accept that you have failed and give yourself an implicit license to abandon your newfound Whole Brain Diet Lifestyle. If you have a short-term relapse, do not let it become a longer-term failure.

Pick yourself up and renew your intention to reclaim the healthier lifestyle you have chosen to adopt. For many people, whether it is quitting smoking, losing weight or any other behavioral change that requires significant effort, going back to old routines happens and is to be expected. Multiple attempts to change may be required, but if you want it badly enough and persevere, you can change your lifestyle permanently. The Whole Brain Diet Lifestyle plan gives you many options to choose from if your initial attempts at change are not successful.

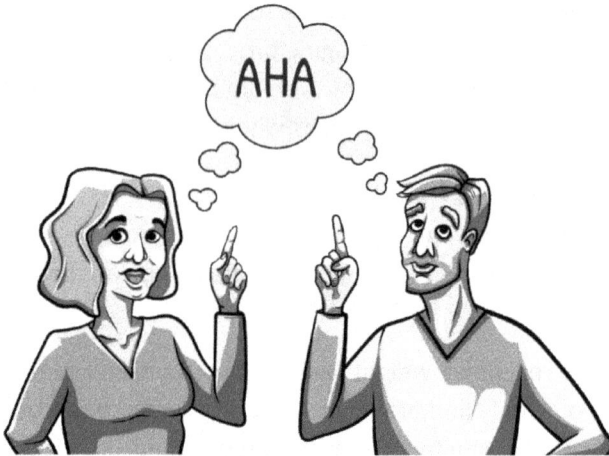

- Make an unbreakable pledge to yourself to activate a contingency plan when you gain more weight than your pre-set limit. This makes weight control easier by minimizing the depletion of your mental energy and your willpower and preserving it for those times when it is more critical to use. Certainty and routine make your brain happy; give it what it wants!
- A daily weigh-in may seem excessive, but it is not. If you catch a weight gain when it is still small, then only small, easy adjustments are needed to lose the weight. This may seem like common sense, but many of us forget and ignore this valuable advice.

Part 5:

Concluding Thoughts

Chapter 21: Implementation Strategy

You need to recognize and accept that you are about to embark on a journey with no end. You must understand that the weight situation you find yourself in right now is the result of many years of following a different, less optimal style of living. It did not evolve overnight, so expecting a rapid resolution to this issue is not only unrealistic but its counterproductive.

Affecting fundamental change takes time, effort and perseverance. Having reasonable expectations is an important prerequisite to nurture the patience needed for real change to take place. You must persevere through the challenges and obstacles you meet on your path to lasting, dietary lifestyle transformation.

An overarching objective is that you want to start with changes that are small, less burdensome and doable. Choose steps that are not too overwhelming, but encourage you to prepare you for the changes that make a lasting difference. Start here, then move on to additional areas. Characteristics of highly desirable, initial behavioral changes are that they:

- are fairly easy to do
- are not central to your core being
- are not disruptive to other family members
- start to reward you quickly
- are without negative, unintended consequences
- can be followed both at home and work

Stage 1: Use the Take 5 Technique

The Take 5 technique satisfies all of the key criteria outlined as being most important in selecting elements of the Whole Brain Diet Lifestyle plan for early adoption. It can be used by virtually everyone and the costs and burden of using it are very small.

Stage 2: Preparing the Mind and Body

Prepare your mind and body by:

- increasing your physical activity, specifically engaging in more exercise
- getting more sleep that's both higher in quality and longer in duration

- spending more time mitigating and managing your stress

These three activities increase your mental energy which increases your will, resolve and self-control, all characteristics that facilitate behavioral change. Make incremental changes that are not too difficult.

Stage 3: Prepare Your Social Environment and Support Systems
Configure your social environment and your relationships to support your quest for lifestyle change. Specifically:

- create a mission statement that reflects your overarching goals for behavior change.
- make a private and public pledge of your intention to change.
- solicit your partner/friends/colleagues to support you and even better enlist one or more of them to join you on your quest to transform your lifestyle.
- set up a reward system with incentives and penalties to support your intentions and increase your motivation to change.

Stage 4: Change Your Environment & Utilize the Power of Your Subconscious
Your environment, physically and psychologically, has a powerful influence on your thoughts, feelings and behaviors. You should:

- start to use all of the tools and tactics recommended in Chapter 11 that you feel you can do and sustain long-term.
- employ the power of the tactics described in the chapter on embodied cognition (Chapter 17).

Stage 5: Psychological Tools and Tactics
Implement the advice given in the chapter on psychological barriers (Chapter 9) and in the chapter on compassion (Chapter 16). These aids may be a little more difficult to use, but they can be extremely beneficial in the long-run to facilitate fundamental change.

Stage 6: Practice the Lifestyle, Be Patient and Persevere
By Stage 6, you are engaged in practicing your new dietary lifestyle. Continue to use the tools and tactics you have chosen for at least three months, long enough for them to become internalized and routine. If you

are satisfied with your progress, keep going. If you are not satisfied, re-read the book and reconfigure the elements of your plan by adding new features and/or eliminating others that were not working for you.

If you follow the implementation plan outlined in this chapter, your odds of success, of achieving permanent, long-term, dietary lifestyle transformation are markedly increased.

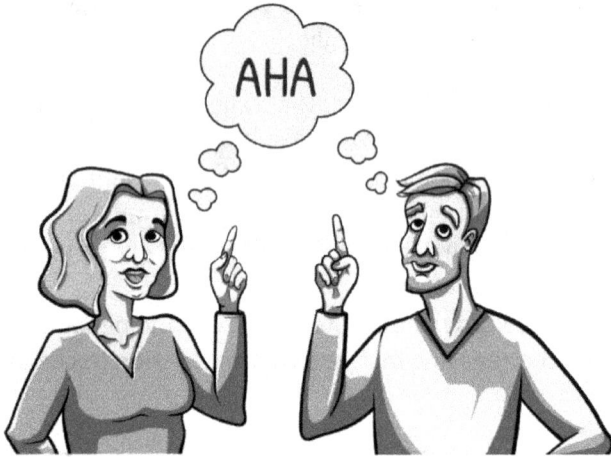

- Following an overall strategy for implementing the Whole Brain Diet Lifestyle plan can materially increase your odds of successfully achieving the lifestyle transformation that you desire.
- Apply your judgment to decide the sequence in which to implement the Whole Brain Diet Lifestyle plan that you feel is likely to work best for you.

Chapter 22 - Whole Brain Diet Lifestyle and Feeling "Hangry"

Being hangry is not a fatal condition, but this doesn't make it any less bothersome.

Several years ago, a new word sprang into the public consciousness and became a catch phrase. The word is "hangry," and while many of you have heard of it, few really know much about it.

What is Hangry?

First, let's be clear. Hanger, what you feel when you become hangry, is a real physiological state with potentially very consequential psychological and behavioral effects.[1] When you have not eaten for an extended period of time and/or you are under sustained physical or mental stress, your blood sugar level runs down. Glucose is the simple sugar your brain uses for fuel (i.e. energy). When the brain senses that its supply of glucose is running low, it responds automatically. Your brain releases hormones to stimulate your hunger and to activate a bodily response that produces more glucose.[2] At the same time that your brain releases the ghrelin hormone that stimulates your hunger, it simultaneously releases stress hormones (like cortisol and adrenaline.)[3] The combination of your hunger and these stress hormones make you feel irritable, cranky and angry, i.e., hangry. It is this combination of hunger and anger that creates the hangry state, and this unleashes a host of negative unintended consequences.

Is Being Hangry Good or Bad?

You might ask, does being hangry serve any positive or productive purpose? Well, it turns out that hangry feelings are favored by evolution as promoting survival, i.e., preservation of the self. In the days of pre-human hominids and early Homo sapiens, food sources were scarce. Individuals who felt hanger were more likely to get their fair share (or more) of the energy sources (i.e. food) available and thereby were more likely to live long enough to procreate and help to perpetuate the species.[4] So evolution has favored those who experience a hangry state. Even today, in an era with readily abundant and accessible food (at least in much of the developed world), the imprint that causes hanger remains in our brain and still generates these feelings, although the positive benefits are diminished.

In the modern world, being hangry has mostly negative consequences. Your hangry feelings spill over and affect those you interact with, whether friends, family or your colleagues. Hanger reduces your ability to control your emotions and makes you more likely to act in socially inappropriate ways.[5] You are less friendly to those around you, and they often respond in kind to you. Hanger is not truly contagious, but the negative emotions it arouses can spread to those around you.

It is, however, not those socially inappropriate acts that have the potential for the greatest and most consequential negative effects. It is the impact that hanger has on how we think, how we engage in complex, mentally challenging activities, how creative we are and very importantly, on our assessment of risk.

Simply put, feeling hangry disrupts your thinking, your focus and your ability to concentrate. At the same time, it makes you more likely to take risks that you would normally avoid.[6] Therefore, never make really important decisions, when feeling hangry. Not only is the quality of your thinking and your analytical capabilities degraded, you are more likely to make rash, poorly reasoned decisions.

Hanger also exacerbates how we react to stimuli in our environment. Whether it is someone talking, chewing gum in the cubicle next to yours or playing the radio a bit too loud. When you feel hangry, these stimuli feel more acute, more annoying.[7] This encourages you to confront a colleague, a neighbor or your partner over something that ordinarily would bother you only a little. Some psychologists have even speculated that acts of violence about seemingly minor provocations (like road rage or parking space disputes) are much more likely among those feeling hangry.[8]

Physiologically, hanger causes us to experience food cravings more often and more intensely.[9] Combined with its lessening of self-control, hanger leads to overeating and bingeing, often on high-sugar foods.

In the 21st century, hanger remains, but has lost its evolutionary advantages, and all that remains are the residual negative byproducts. Is the control of hanger a lost cause? The answer is no, the means to avoid or minimize it are known, but not so easy to follow. Most of us still fall prey to feeling hangry and to the effects associated with that state of being.

How to Avoid Becoming Hangry

To avoid feeling hangry, you can simply eat something every two to three hours.[10] Further, if you feel hangry and respond to its urgent call for food, you can eat a whole grain and/or high-fiber snack (like fruits/or veggies) that not only satisfies your hunger, but also prevents a blood sugar spike and a repeat of the cycle later in the day.[11]

The real deterrent to adopting these tactics is that too many of us are already overweight or obese, and we deal with this by using traditional, or even worse, fad diets. These diets, which are typically based on some type of deprivation, keep our bodies in a continual low-level state of hunger with an accompanying low, but real, hangry feelings. These low-level hangry feelings still exert negative effects on your self-control, your emotional state and your decision making. The solution is to avoid diets and go down the path of long-term diet lifestyle transformation. The Whole Brain Diet Lifestyle provides the natural solution to avoid hanger and to minimize its negative consequences when you do experience it.

In summary, actively take charge of your brain, create healthy habits that replace the old automatic, negative ones that used to rule your life. Then you are in position to avoid feelings of hanger altogether or to recognize its emergence at an early stage where you can best mitigate its effects.

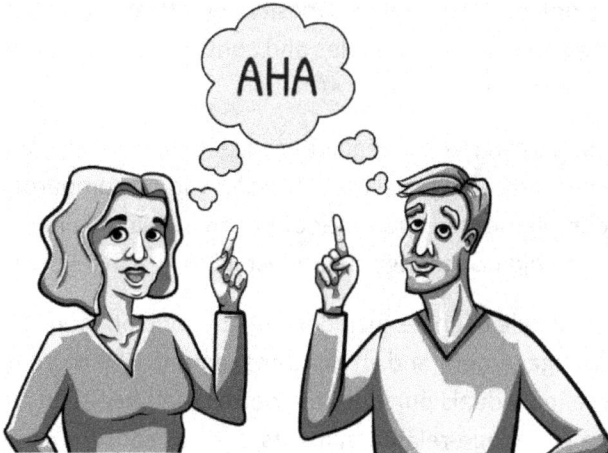

- Being hangry once served an important evolutionary purpose, but today it is merely a distraction with real negative consequences.
- Dieting is a primary cause of becoming hangry; following the Whole Brain Diet Lifestyle provides a natural deterrent to avoid it.

Chapter 23: Final Thoughts

This book provides a comprehensive and practical array of tools and tactics you can use to transform your dietary lifestyle, health and life. Following the Whole Brain Diet Lifestyle not only improves your health and well-being, as a natural byproduct you lose weight.

By now you should have had a chance to identify those specific elements of the Whole Brain Diet Lifestyle plan that appeal to you and which you believe you can adopt and integrate into your life. The Whole Brain Diet Lifestyle plan is not a "one size fits all," it presents more of a buffet of tools and tactics for you to select from. You should select a particular configuration of elements to try. If you do not find yourself moving toward your lifestyle transformation goals and acceptable weight loss after several months, go back and pick a new assortment of elements and try them. The incredible array of choices the Whole Brain Diet Lifestyle plan provides puts you in charge.

To review why lifestyle change is so important and can be so consequential to your life by ask the question, "Why does implementing positive, healthy lifestyle changes really matter?" Being greatly overweight or obese has negative effects on your body and your mind. Obesity is now thought to add as much as 10 years to the cellular age of your body and your organs.[1] Your brain is one of those organs. Obesity in your later years may degrade your thinking and analytical abilities and contribute to the onset of brain disorders such as Alzheimer's.

Lifestyle changes can make a real difference in how we age and our likelihood of getting an age-related disease. A study compared a group of people who implemented a number of positive, healthy, lifestyle changes with those who did not change their lifestyle over a five-year period.

The healthy lifestyle changes included weight control, moderate exercise, active social engagement and stress management. The more of these behaviors the individuals pursued, the better their health at the cellular level and the fewer age-related ailments, such as cancer and dementia, they were expected to have.[2]

Not only will implementing healthy lifestyle changes have a profoundly positive impact on your physical and brain health, but also on your mental and emotional health. If that is not worth the effort of striving to make behavioral changes in your life, including your diet lifestyle, I do not know what would be.

Always remember that your brain is the master of your behavior and that YOU are the master of your brain!

Chapter Notes

Prologue

[1] *"Obesity and Overweight,"www.cdc.gov/nchs/fastats/overwt.htm*; CDC "Obesity in the US,"http://frac.org/initiatives/hunger-and-obesity/obesity-in-the-us/, Food Research and Action Center

[2] "Obesity & Diabetes Double the Risk of Heart Failure, www.sciencedaily.com/releases/2009/05/090530094510.htm; *6.4.09 "Virtual Epidemic, "www.completerx.com/tag/virtual-epidemic*

[3] "Why 95% of Dieters Gain the Weight Back, "www.healthread.net/why-dieters-regain-leibel.htm

[4] Daniel Kahneman, *Thinking Fast and Slow,* Farrar, Straus & Giroux 2011

Introduction

[1] Dr. Andrew Weil, *Healthy Aging,* Knopf Doubleday,1.2.07, pg. 22,; Rudolph Tanzi & Deepak Chopra *Super Brain,*, Random House, 2012, pg./ 170

[2] Richard Brodie,*Virus of the Mind,* Hay House, 11.7.09 pg.59

[3] David DiSalvo, *What Makes Your Brain Happy and Why You Should Do the Opposite,* Prometheus Books, 11/22.11 pg.138; Richard Brodie,*"Virus of the Mind,"* 11.7.09, pg.83

[4] Richard Brodie,*Virus of the Mind,* 11.7.09

[5] Nevin Scrimshaw, "World Problems, www.encyclopedia.com/topic/Food.aspx, 2008

[6] David Linden,*The Compass of Pleasure,* Penguin Books,4.24.12, pg.83,

[7] Dr. Andrew Weil, *Healthy Aging,* Knopf DFoubleday pg.70

[8] Jane Brody, "Personal Health," The NY Times, 10.23.12

[9] "Bitter Taste Identifies Poisons in Food, "www.eurekalert.org/pub_releases/2006-09/mcsc-bti091206.php, 9.18.06

[10] "Glycemic Index," http://nutritondata.self.com/topics/glycemic-index; Mayo Clinic Staff, "Glycemic Index Diet: what's behind the claims, www.mayoclinic.org/healthy-lifestyle-nutrition-and-healthy-eatng/in-depth/glycemic/index-diet/art

[11] David Linden,*The Compass of Pleasure, 4.24.12,* pg.83

[12] Kelly Traver, *The Program: The Brain-Smart Approach to the Healthiest You,* Simon and Schuster, 2009, pg.39

13 Drew Desilver, "How Americas Diet Has Changed Over Time," www.pewresearch.org, 12.13.16

[14] Daniel Kahneman, *Thinking Fast and Slow,* 2011, pg.4-20

[15] Daniel Kahneman, *Thinking Fast and Slow*, 2011, pg.21

[16] Rudolph Tanzi & Deepak Chopra, *Super Brain,*, 2012, pg.256

Chapter 1: Cravings & the Take 5 Technique

[1] *"Sugar and Dopamine: The Link Between Sweets and Addiction"*   *wellness* *retreatrecovery.com*

[2] *http://healthvibed.com/relaxation-101-how-to-activate-the-pns/*

[3]*Ana Sandoiv, "Stressed Out? Try Talking to Yourself in the Third Person," Medical News Today, 7.30.17*

[4] *Robert Sapolsky, Behave, Penguin Press, 2017*

[5] *Robert Sapolsky, Behave, pg. 67, Penguin Press, 2017*

[6] *Robert Sapolsky, Behave, pg. 67, Penguin Press, 2017*

[7] *Caroline Beaton, "The Work Humans Are Wired to Do," Psychology Today, 5.23.17*

[8] *From an interview with Angela Duckworth, Heleo.com*

Chapter 2: More Take 5 Applications

[1] *Jill Bolte Taylor, Butler Univ. commencement speech, 5.9.16*

[2] *Eudaimonic well-being is based on seeking meaning and self-realization as opposed to seeking pleasure and reward*

Chapter 3: Why is Weight Loss so Difficult

[1] "Obesity & Overweight," *www.cdc.gov/nchs/fastats/overwt.htm, CDC.*

[2] "Obesity in theU.S.,"http://frac.org/initiatives/hunger-and-obesity/obesity-in-the-us/, Food Research and Action Center

[3] "Why 95% of Dieters Gain the Weight Back",www.healthread.net/why-dieters-regain-leibel.htm

[4] www.foxnews.com/health/2015/03/13/why-exercise-and-diet-changes-may-not-be-enough-to-treat-obesity/

[5] *Sandra Aamodt, "Why Dieting Doesn't Usually Work," https://ted.com*

[6] *"How fat cells work and why it's impossible to "burn" them off, "www.qz.com/654547/everything-you-need-to-know-about-fat-cells,*

[7] *"Why the Eat Less Move More Approach Often Fails,"* www.psychologytoday.com/blog/contempporary-psychoanalysis-in-action/201502/why-the-eat-less-move-more-approach-often-fails

[8] *"The Week" Magazine, January 15, 2016, pg.6*

[9] *ABC News report, 2/10/16*

Chapter 4: How and Why the Whole Brain Diet Lifestyle Works
[1] Daniel Pink, *Drive,* Penguin Publishing Group, 2009

[2] Daniel Pink, *Drive,* 2009, pgs. 70-71

[3] Definition of "mindfulness" found via Google search: attribution unknown

[4] www.theguardian.com/science/neurophilosophy/2016/Nov/23/obesity-alters-brain-structure and function.

[5] "Neural Basis for Cravings"www.psypostng/2016/12/neuroscientist-brain-reacts-similarly-drugs-high-calorie-food-46913

Chapter 5: The Concept and Role of Mental Energy
[1] my interpretation and extrapolation of the definition of mental energy found in: www.thefreedictionary.com/mental+ene; www.audioenglish.org/dictionary/mental_energy.htmrgy;

[2] Julia Layton, "Is it true that if you do anything for three weeks it will become a habit?" http://science.howstuffworks.com/life/form-a-habit2.htm

[3] **http:///www.stanford.edu/.../Job,%20Walton,%20Bernecker,..;**
"Ego Depletion," http://en.wikipedia.org/wiki/Ego_depletion

Chapter 6: Neuroplasticity & Behavior Change
[1] "Neuroplasticity," *en.wikipedia.org/wiki/Neuroplasticity*

[2] *"Neuroplasticity," en.wikipedia.org/wiki/Neuroplasticity*

[3] *Rudy Tanzi & Deepak* Chopra, *Super Brain,* pg.26

[4] *"Five Ways to Rewire Your Brain," mindbodygreen.com/0-111762/5-*

ways-to-rewire...; Dr. Michael Mezernich, Soft-Wired (How the New Science

of Brain Plasticity Can Change Your Life) , 10.14.13, pgs. 41,46, 150,174,212

Chapter 7: A "Lite" Approach to Life
[1] http://www.thefreedictionary.com/lightness

Chapter 8: Setting New Goals and Creating New Habits
[1] *Oxford Dictionary, www.oed.com*

[2] David McRaney, "You are not so smart," 11.6.12, pgs. 191, 193, 195, 217

[3] "Journal of Positive Psychology," Volume 7, Number 1, January 2012, pages 7-71

[4] "Nutrition Reviews," Volume 64, Issue 12, pages 518-531, 12/2006

[5] David DiSalvo, "What Makes Your Brain Happy and Why You Should Do the Opposite,"

11.22.11, pages 70, 225-226;

[6] Daniel Kahneman, "Thinking Fast and Slow," 2011, page 128

[7] Kelly Traver, "The Program: The Brain Smart Approach to the Healthiest You," 2009, page 30

[8] Rudolph Tanzi & Deepak Chopra, "Super Brain: Getting Started Now-Workbook," 2012, page 26

[9] http://www.swc.osu.edu/healthy-eating-active-living/weight management/stages-of-change

[10] "Why Diets Fail," 11.18.2011

[11] Rudolph Tanzi & Deepak Chopra, "Super Brain: Getting Started Now-Workbook," 2012, page 58; www.en.wikipedia.org/goal_setting

Chapter 9: Psychological Barriers

[1] Richard Brodie, *Virus of the Mind*, 11.7.09 pg. 69-70

[2] "Virus of the Mind," Richard Brodie, 11.7.09, pg. 84

[3] "Virus of the Mind," Richard Brodie, 11.7.09, pg.18

[4] www.serendip.brynmawr.edu/bb/kinser/Structure1

[5] www.serendip.brynmawr.edu/bb/kinser/Structure1

[6] David McRaney, *You Are Not So Smart*, Penguin Random House, *11.6.12*, pg.23,66

[7] Daniel Kahneman, *Thinking Fast and Slow*, 2011, pg. 415.

Wayne Dyer, "Excuses Begone," Hay House, 1.11.11, pg.22

[8] David DiSalvo, *What Makes Your Brain Happy and Why You Should Do the Opposite*, pg.32,52

[9] "What Makes Your Brain Happy and Why You Should Do the Opposite," David DiSalvo, 11.22.11 pg.83-85; Daniel Kahneman, *Thinking Fast and Slow*, 2011, pg. 21

[10] Wayne Dyer, *Excuses Begone*, 1.1.11, pg.188

[11] John Ratey, *Spark-The Revolutionary Science of Exercise and the Brain*, Little Brown & Co. 2008

[12] Wayne Dyer, *Excuses Begone,* Wayne Dyer,1.1.11, pg.22

[13] www.serendip.brynmawr.edu/bb/kinser/Structure1

[14] Helen Kollias, "www.precisionnutrition.com/how-to-change-behaviour

15 Based on the ideas of Professor John Norcross of the U. of Scranton

[16] David McRaney, *You Are Not So Smart*, 11.6.12, pg.205,231,235; Daniel Amen, *Change Your Brain, Change Your Body*, Penguin Random House, 12.28.10, pg. 270; Norman Cousins, *Head First-The Biology of Hope and the Healing Power of the Human Spirit*, Dutton pg.18

[17] "Self-Sabotage Behavior," www.life-with-*confidence*.com/self-sabotage-behavior

[18] Daniel Kahneman, *Thinking Fast and Slow*, 2011, pg. 257

[19] Amy Cuddy, *Presence*, Little Brown & Co., 11.3.15

[20] Leo Babauta, "Wake Up: A Guide to Living Your Life Consciously, "zenhabits.net/wake-up-a-guide-to-living-your-life-consciously

[21] Waldman & Newberg, *How God Changes Your Brain*," Penguin Random House, 5.23.10

[22] Daniel Kahneman, *Thinking Fast and Slow*, 2011, pg.367

[23] David McRaney, *You Are Not So Smart*, 11.6.12, pg.191;"Why Diets Fail," "The Week Magazine," 11/18/2011

[24] "http://serendip.brynmawr.edu/exchange/node/3923, (based on "Train Your Mind, Change Your Brain", by Sharon Begley)

[25] Charles Duhigg, *The Power of Habit*, Random House, 2012

[26] Kelly McGonigal, *The Willpower Instinct: How Self-Control Works, Why It Matters, and What You Can Do to Get More of It*, Penguin Random House, 2014; "www.nytimes.com/2011/08/21/magazine/do-you-suffer-from-decision-fatigue

[27] Daniel Kahneman, *Thinking Fast and Slow*, 2011, pg.43; Kelly McGonigal, *The Willpower Instinct*, 2011

[28] Roy Baumeister & Jon Tierney, *Willpower-Rediscovering the Greatest Human Strength*, Penguin Random House, 8.28.12

[29]"Kelly McGonigal quoted in "Psychology Today," July/Sugust 2012

[30] Kelly McGonigal,*The Willpower Instinct*, 2014

[31] Adam Gurlick,"Media Multitaskers Pay Mental Price, Stanford Study Shows," Stanford University News, 8/24/09

[32] Wayne Dyer, *Excuses Begone*, 1.1.11, pg. 89-91; Rudolph Tanzi & Deepak Chopra, *Super Brain*, 11.12 pg.98

[33] Rudolph Tanzi & Deepak Chopra, *Super Brain*, 11.12, pg.136

[34] Stress Management: Breathing Exercises for Relaxation," "www.*webmd.com/stress/stress-management-breathing-exercises*

[35] Exercise and Stress: Get Moving to Manage Stress," www.mayoclinic.com/health/exercise-and-stress/SR00036

[36] David DiSalvo, *What Makes Your Brain Happy and Why You Should Do the Opposite*, 11.22.11, pg.221

[37] "Self-Awareness," http://www.change-management-coach.com/self-awareness.html

Chapter 10: Social Barriers

[1] David McRaney, *What Makes Your Brain Happy and Why You Should Do the Opposite*, Prometheus Books, 11.15.11 pg.110-111

[2] David McRaney, *You Are Not So Smart*," 11.6.12, pg.243-244

[3] David DiSalvo, *What Makes Your Brain Happy and Why You Should Do the Opposite*, 11.22.11, pg. 164

[4] Waldman & Newberg, *How God Changes Your Brain*, 5.23.10

[5] Roxanne Dryden-Edwards, "Emotional Eating," http://www.Medicinenet.com/emotional_eating/article.htm;

"Emotional Eating and Stress Craving," www.helpguide/Org/life/emotional_eating_stress_craving.htm

Chapter 11: Physical Barriers

[1] Some of the thoughts and tips in this chapter are based on my own personal observation and common sense, unless otherwise noted.

[2] Common sense suggests that shopping on the weekend is less stressful and less hurried

[3] "Our Best 75 Weight-loss Tips," Woman's Day.com/health-fitness

[4] "Wellness Letter," U. of California, Berkeley, 4/1/12

[5] "Top 10 Make or Break Diet Moments," Fitness Magazine, Amanda Vogel, 10/2/12

[6] David Zinczenko, author and editor-in-chief , Men's Health magazine

[7] Wayne Dyer, *Excuses Begone*," 1.1.11, pg.19-20

[8] Consistent with basic premise of book to construct barriers to reduce food/snack accessibility

[9] Consistent with basic premise of book to construct barriers to reduce food/snack accessibility

[10] Consistent with basic premise of book to construct barriers to reduce food/snack accessibility

[11] Suggested by a passage in "Mindwise," Nicholoas Epley, pgs.68-69

[12] "Weird Colors: Colors Can Help You Lose Weight," health.yahoo.net, 8/21/12

[13] Baumeister & Tierney *Willpower-Redsicovering the Greatest Human Strength*," 8.28.12; Kelly McGonigal, *The Willpower Instinct*, 2011

[14] Dr. David Katz, "The No Diet Approach," Webmd.com; oprah.com/health," 8/09; Rudolph Tanzi & Deepak Chopra, *Super Brain-The Workbook*, 2012, pg.81

[15] "The perils of skipping breakfast," The Week Magazine, August 9, 2013, pg.18

[16] 10 New Weight Loss Myths & Facts," "shine.yahoo.com/healthy-living; Baumeister & Tierney, *Willpower-Rediscovering the Greatest Human Strength*," 8.28.12

[17] Our Best 75 Weight-loss Tips," WomansDay.com/health-fitness; "shine.yahoo.com/photos/25-healthy-tips," Yahoo.com, 3/10/13

[18] "20 Ways to Speed Up Your Metabolism," Heather Bauer, "Redbook Magazine," 2/22/12

[19] "Life-long Weight Loss 'Secrets'," health.yahoo.net/articles/weight-loss

[20] Shine.yahoo.com/healthy," Heather Kolich, 11/23/12

[21] www.ajcn.nutrition.org/content/82/1/222S.full

"Losing Weight and Keeping It Off," www.cdc.gov/healthyweight/losing_weight/keepingitoff.html.

[22] Dr. M. Oz,"Skinny Gene Discovery,"For Women First Magazine,", 3/26/12," ; N. Swaminanthan,"How to Save Your Brain," "Psychology Today," Jan/Feb 2012

[23] "Wellness Letter," U. Of California, Berkeley, Vol. 28, Issue 11, Summer, 2012"Glycemic Index Diet," US News, 11/19/11

[24] Cynthia Sass, "Shine from Yahoo!, " Shape Magazine; " A. Sansone, "Women's 8 Biggest Eating Mistakes,"womansday.com/healthy-living

[25] "Shine from Yahoo," "Readers Digest Magazine," 1/17/12

[26] Heather Bauer,"20 Ways to Speed Up Your Metabolism," 'Redbook Magazine," 2/22/12: "Snack Smart," AARP Magazine, 4/12

[27] Kelly Traver, *The Program: The Brain-Smart Approach to the Healthiest You*, 2009, pg.132

[28] One of the most basic points of this book is to limit accessibility

[29] "Women's 8 Biggest Eating Mistakes," A. Sansone, WomansDay.com/healthyliving,

[30] Dr. David Katz, "Life-long Weight Loss Secrets,"Oprah.com/health," 8/09; " health.yahoo.net/articles/weight-loss

[31] The No Diet Approach,"Webmd.com; "Slim for Life: 10 strategies to Lose Fat and Keep It off," "Fitness Magazine"

[32]"Slim for life: 10 Strategies to Lose Fat and Keep It Off," Fitness Magazine and other common sense strategies

[33] "Portion Size Research," "www.cdc.gov/nccdphp/dnpa/nutrition/pdf/portion_size_research; www.choosemyplate.gov/weight-management-calories/weight-management/better-choices/decrease-portions.html

[34] Dr. David Katz,"Oprah.com/health," 8/09; "eatingwell.com/nutrition"

[35]www.wikihow.com/Control-Food-Portions; Maura Shenker, " Three Benefits of Eating Smaller Portions,"www.livestrong.com/article/297709-small-plate-diet/

[36]"Weird Colors: Colors Can Help You Lose Weight," health.yahoo.net, 8/21/12; "Think More, Eat Less," U. of California, "Wellness Letter," 3/13

[37] Rudolph Tanzi & Deepak Chopra, *Super Brain*," 2012

[38]shine.yahoo.com/photos/25-healthy-tips," Yahoo.com, 3/10/13

[39] "The Week" Magazine, 3/4/16, page 8

[40] Allison Aubrey, "Circadian Surprise: How Our Body Clock Helps Shape Our Waistlines," www.npr.org/blogs/thesalt/2015/03/10/389596946/circadian-surprise

[41] "Weight Loss: Why you should put up a mirror in the kitchen," www.spring.org.uk, 3.19.16

[42] "Regular Mealtimes - The Basics," http://nutrition.getfit.com/tips/regular-eating

[43]Based on personal author's personal observation and common sense

[44]Snack Smart," AARP Magazine, 4/12

[45] Baumeister & Tierney, *Willpower-Rediscovering the Greatest Human Strength*,; "How to Save Your Brain," Psychology Today, Jan./Feb 2012

[46] Kelly Traver,*The Program: The Brain-Smart Approach to the Healthiest You*, 2009, pg.291-293; Clockwork Orange....," "Psychology Today," pg.44-45, Jan/Feb. 2013

[47] Malia Wollan, "Failure to Lunch,"NY Times Magazine, 2/28/16

[48] Stephan Guyenet, *The Hungry Brain*, Flatiron Books 2017, pg.158

Chapter 12: Genes and Memes
[1] Rudolph Tanzi & Deepak Chopra, "Super Genes," Random House, 2015

[2] Richard Brodie, *Virus of the Mind*, 1996

Chapter 13: Exercise
[1] Kelly Traver, *The Program-The Brain-Smart Approach to the Healthiest You*, 2009, pg.361

[2] Kelly Traver, *The Program-The Brain-Smart Approach to the Healthiest You*, pg.54-56; Andrew Weil, *Healthy Aging*, 1.2.07, pg.178-181

[3] "A Stronger Heart May Keep Your Brain Young," www.health.harvard.edu/blog/a-stronger-heart-may-keep-your-brain-young

[4] Gretchen Reynolds, "Exercise May Fend Off Depression," NY Times,11/22/16

[5] "Which is Better for Weight Loss-Cutting Calories or Increasing Exercise?" "www.mayoclinic.com/health/weight-loss/AN01619; "www.nytimes.com/2010/04/18/magazine/18exercise-t.html?pagewanted=all&_r=0

[6] John Swartzberg,"Exercise Because it Feels Good," Wellness Letter, 1/2013, pg.3

[7] *http:/fithabits.com/21-habit-quotes-that-will-inspire-you-to-lose-weight*

[8] Susan Scutti, *"Yes, sitting too long can kill you, even if you exercise," CNN, 9.11.17*

[9]"Start Your Own Exercise regimen & Stick to It,""www.wikihow.com/Start-Your-Own-Exercise-Regimen-and-Stick-to-It; "5 Ways to Keep Up Your Workout Motivation, "www.huffingtonpost.com/2011/10/01/5-ways-to-keep-up-your-workout-motivation_n_988515.html

[10] http://www.mayoclinic.com/health/exercise/SM00109

[11] "Exercise Can Extend Your Life as Much as Five Years," www.sciencedaily.com/releases/2012/12/121211082810.htm;

"Add 6 Years to Your Life by Jogging,"www.hivehealthmedia.com/add-6-years-to-your-life-jogging/

[12]*http:/fithabits.com/21-habit-quotes-that-will-inspire-you-to-lose-weight*

[13]"Lifestyle Activity-it adds up and pays off, Wellness Letter,"University of California, Berkley, June 2013, page 6

[14]The 10 Most Misunderstood Diet & Fitness Strategies," Shine from Yahoo, Shape Magazine, 6/29/2012

[15] "How Much Exercise Do You Really Need-Less Than You Think" www.health.harvard.edu/blog/how-much-exercise-do-you-really-need-less-than-you-think

[16] John Swartzberg, "Exercise Because it Feels Good," Wellness Letter, 1/2013, pg.3: " The Benefits of Exercising Outdoors," well.blogs.nytimes.com/2013/02/21/the-benefits-of-exercising-outdoors/

[17] "Why Exercising Makes Us Happier,"blog.bufferapp.com/why-exercising-makes-us-happier; "The Benefits of outdoor Exercise Confirmed, "www.sciencedaily.com/releases/2011/02/110204130607.htm

[18] Gretchen Reynolds, "The Benefits of Exercising Before Breakfast, "www.well.blogs.nytimes.com/2000/12/15-phys-ed-the-benefits-of-exercising-before-breakfast, 12.15.2010; Lisa Freedman, "When to Eat Breakfast-Before or After a Workout?"

www.mensfitness.com/nutrition-when-to-eat-breakfast-before-or-after-a-workout

[19] "Stressed at Work-Try a Lunchtime Walk," mobile.nytimes.com/blogs/2015/01/21/stressed-at-work-try-a-lunchtime-walk......

Chapter 14: Stress

[1] http://www.helpguide.org/mental/stress_signs.htm

[2] "Ways Stress Can Make You Fat," www.cheatsheet.com/health-fitness/ways-stress-can-make-you-fat

[3] Baumeister & Tierney *Willpower-Rediscovering the Greatest Human Strength*," 2011

[4] "Reasons Nature Can Heal Your Mind," www.spring.org.uk/2014/07/10-reasons-nature-can-heal-your-mind

[5] www.healinggateways.com/Reduce-Stress; "How to Relieve Stress", *www.audiotranscription.org/how-to-relieve-stress*

[6] Daniel Kahneman, "Thinking Fast and Slow," 2011, pg. 416

[7] Emma Seppala, *The Happiness Track*," HarperCollins, 2016 pgs. 48-49

Chapter 15: Sleep

[1] Heather Kolich, "Life-long Weight Loss 'Secrets'," "shine.yahoo/healthy," 11.23.12; health.yahoo.net/articles/weight-loss; Tara Parker-Pope, "Lost Sleep Can Lead to Weight Gain," NY Times, 3/19/13, Section D4

[2] "Shine from Yahoo," 'Readers Digest magazine," 1/17/12

"News You Can Use," US News, 7/7/12; eatingwell.com/nutrition

[4] Carolyn Gregoive, "Sleep Health Benefits: A Good Night's Rest Boosts Benefits of a Heart-Healthy Lifestyle", Huffington-Post.com 7/3/13

[5] "What is the Magic Sleep Number," www.health.harvard.edu/blog-what-is-the-magic-sleep-number

[6] http://en.wikipedia.org/wiki/Segmented_sleep; Paul Spector, "Why You Might Have Trouble Sleeping," http://www.huffingtonpost.com/paul-spector-md/why-you-might-have-troubl_b_1883811.html

[7] www.ventures.com/business-guide/crosscuttngs/mir; http://en.wikipedia.org/wiki/Human_multitasking

Chapter 16: Compassion

[1] "Mother Teresa Quotes,

"http://www.goodreads.com/author/quotes/8305.Mother_Teresa?page=2

[2] from the Beatles song, "The End"

[3] based on a quote appearing in "The Week" magazine, page 15, July 19, 2013

[4] manifestexcellence.com/.../the-health-benefits-of-kindness-compassion-a...; www.psychologicalscience.org/index.../the-compassionate-mind.html.

"A Guide to Cultivating Compassion in Your Life with 7 Practices, "zenhabits.net/a-guide-to-cultivating-compassion-in-your-life-with-7-prac...

[5] Adam Grant, Give and Take, Penguin Random House, 2013, pages 179-185

[6] Emma Seppala, The Happiness Track, 2016, pgs. 135-139

Chapter 17: Embodied Cognition

[1] "Seindfeld" TV Show, November 18, 1992, Season 4, Episode 11

[2] Thalma Lobel, "Sensation (The New Science of Physical Intelligence"), Atria Books, 2014

[3] Thalma Lobel, "Sensation (The New Science of Physical Intelligence"), Atria Books, 2014

[4] Meir, Schnali, Schwarz & Bargh, "Embodied in Social Psychology," https://dornsife.usc.edu/assets/sites/780/docs/12_topics_meier_et_al_embodiement, 1/24/2011

[5] Thalma Lobel, "Sensation (The New Science of Physical Intelligence"), Atria Books, 2014

[6] "Remember Hard, But Think Softly: Metaphorical Effects of Sitting on a hard Surface",www.ncbi.nim.nih.gov,

[7] Spence, Harrar & Fiszman, "Assessing the impact of the tableware and other contextual variables on multisensory flavor perception, "https://flavourjournal:biomeicalcentral.com/articles/10.1186/2044-7248-1-7

[8] www.futureoffood.ox.ac.uk/

[9] Glen Nunes, "The Psychology of Color-How Color Affects Human Behavior, "https://feltmagnet.com, 1/10/2017

[10] " 3 Surprising Ways Nature Leads to Success and Joy," "http://fulfillmentrdaily.com/3-surprising-ways-nature-leads-to-success-and-joy

[11] Katherine Derla,"This is How Eating in Front of Mirror Can Help You Lose Weight," www.techtimes.com, 1/05/2016

[12] Nancy Wells, "The openness of a floor plan could affect how much you eat, study says." "www.psypost.org/2017/07/openness-floor-plan-affects-how-much-you-eat,

[13] Sharon Payne, "The Impact of Environment for Shaping Food Intake-Does It Contribute to Obesity," https://wakespace.lib.wfu.edu/bitstream/handle/10339..., May 2010

[14] Thalma Lobel, "Sensation (The New Science of Physical Intelligence")," Atria Books, 2014

[15] Amy Cuddy, *Presence, 11.3.15*

[16] Russ Swan "Watching Imagination in action: Scientists discover what happens in the brain as we daydream and have creative thoughts," https://secured.dailymail.co.uk," 3/10/2016

[17] "Squeezing a Rubber Ball May Boost Creative Thinking" https://psychcentral.com,

Chapter 18: Whole Brain Diet Lifestyle, Take 5 & Parents

[1] "Overweight in Children," American Heart Association,www.heart.org

[2] Eric Carrick,"Biggest Causes of Obesity in Children,

"CheatSheet.com/health, 8.8.17

[3] livescience.com/37703-epigenetics

[4] livescience.com/37703-epigenetics

[5] "Exercise During Pregnancy May Benefit Kids Long Term Health

www.psychologytoday.com/blog/the-athletes-way-201611/exercise-

during-pregnancy-may-benefit-kids-long-term-health

[6] "Mother's High Fast Diet Alters Metabolism of Offspring Leading to

Higher Obesity Risk,"

http://news.yale.edu/2014/01/23/mothers-high-fat-diet-alters

metabolism-of-offspring-leading-higher-obesity-risk

[7] role of parents on children/childhood imprinting

"www.livestrong.com/article/75282-parents-effect-child-behavior/.

"www.eufic.org/article/en/artid/Parental-influence-children-food-

preferences-and-energy-intake/

[8] RudolphTanzi & Deepak Chopra-*Super Brain* re. childhood imprinting,

pg.52

[9] Sugar lights up child's brain reward center,

"ideas.time.com/2012/12/27/what-you-need-

to-know-about-sugar/; "www.psychologytoday.com/blog/you-illuminated/201108/7-things-mcdonald-s-knows- about-your-brain "

[10] "Mistake emotional pain for physical hunger signal",

"www.helpguide.org/life/emotional_eating_stress_cravings.htm.

"www.anonymityone.com/faq102.htm

[11]"www.healthychildren.org/English/ages-stages/baby/crying-

colic/pages/Responding-to-Your-Babys-Cries.aspx.

"Crying and Fussing in an Infant" "www.healthofchildren.com/C/Crying-

and-Fussing-in-an-Infant.html

Chapter 19: Whole Brain Diet Lifestyle Plan Alternative

[1] "Sugar Can Be Addictive, Princeton Scientist Says,"

www.princeton.edu/main/news/archive/S22/88/56G31/index.xml?

section=topstories; "Mood-Food Relationships,"

www.faqs.org/nutrition/Met-Obe/Mood-Food-Relationships.html

[2] "How Much Sugar Do We Eat, "blissfulwriter.com/hubpages/hub/how-

much-sugar-do-we-eat

[3] www.ehow.com/list_7668159_risks_increased-sugar-cunsumption

[4] Katie Moisse, "25,000 U.S. Deaths Linked to Sugary Drinks," ABC News,

3/19/13

[5] "Diet Soda Diabetes Risk,"huffingtonpost.com/2013/02/11/diet-soda-

diabetes-risk; "Side Effects of Diet Soda,"

healthyliving.msn/health-wellness/7-side-effects-of-diet-soda

[6] "Diet Soda Health Risks: Study Says Artificial Sweeteners May Cause

Weight Gain, Deadly Diseases," Huffington-post, 7/11/13

Chapter 20: Thermostatic Weight Control Approach

[1] Kelly Traver, The Program: The Brain-Smart Approach to the Healthiest

You, 2009, pg.346; "shine.yahoo.com/healthy, Heather Kolich, 11/23/12

[2]"How to Trick Yourself into Eating Well," Prevention.com

[3] www.mayoclinic.com/health/positive-thinking/SR00009

4 CNNMoney.com, 7/2012

5 Jessica Smith,"22 Ways to Stay Motivated to Lose Weight,"
shape.com/print/19635

Chapter 22: Final Thoughts

1 "Effects of obesity on the human brain,

"http://brainblogger.com/2016/10/28/effect-of-obesity-on-human-brain

2 "How Changes to your Diet and Exercise Regime Could Transform Your

Cells-and Your Life,Huffingtonpost.com, Amanda Chan, 9.16/13

Appendix: Whole Brain Diet Lifestyle & Feeling 'Hangry'

1 *"The Science Behind Why You Get Hangry,"* "http://www.huffingtonpost.com/life-by-dailyburn-/the-science-behind-why-you-get-hangry_b_9170500.html

2 "What Happens to Your Body When You Are Hangry,"

 http://www.eatthis.com/hangry,

3 "The Science Behind Why You Get Hangry" http://www.huffingtonpost.com/life-by-dailyburn-/the-science-behind-why-you-get-hangry_b_9170500.html

4 "Feeling Hangry? How to Avoid Food-Related Mood Swings,"
"http://www.thealternativedaily.com/hangry-food-mood-swings/

5 "Feeling Hangry? How to Avoid Food-Related Mood Swings,

"http://www.thealternativedaily.com/hangry-food-mood-swings/

6 Justin Caba "Hangry is a Real Thing...," http://www.medicaldaily.com/hangry-real-thing-hunger-pangs-not-only-worsen-your-mood-trigger-risky-behavior-247129

7 Eleanor Morgan, "Stressful Living is Giving Us All Hunger Rage,
"https://munchies.vice.com/articles/stressful-modern-life-is-giving-us-all-hunger-rage

8 Becca Caddy,"Being Hangry is a Real Thing, According to Science,"
http://www.lifehacker.co.uk/2016/01/04/being-hangry-is-a-real-thing-according-to-science

9 Olivia Tarentino, "What Happens to Your Body When You're Hangry,
"http://www.eatthis.com/hangry

10 "The Science Behind Why You Get Hangry," http://www.huffingtonpost.com/life-by-dailyburn-/the-science-behind-why-you-get-hangry_b_9170500.html

11 Todd Van Luling "How to Never Get Hangry Again,"
http://www.huffingtonpost.com/2014/05/01/hangry-what-to-eat_n_5192313.html

About the Author

Ken Derow once worked for the forces of "evil." He enjoyed an almost 40-year career in consumer marketing research, helping large, multinational corporations to expand their wallets while expanding your waistline. He helped to stoke our cravings for Pepperidge Farms Goldfish, Tastykake Krimpets, or any number of other mass-produced ultra-processed junk foods. Those empty calories may have found their way into your house because of his extensive experience in consumer behavior, decision-making and psychology. However, his passion for promoting unhealthful products waned as his own waistline expanded and he partook in his own journey to become more healthful and lose weight. Like many, he struggled to find the right path to balance his craving for junk foods against his conscious desire to consume more healthful choices. He extensively researched brain science, psychology, eating behavior and the basis for the cravings that drive snacking, overeating and bingeing. This research was the basis for the *TAKE 5* book and the diet lifestyle plan he developed allowed him to achieve a very significant weight loss and maintain it permanently. The huge amount of secondary research Ken conducted into consumer behavior and decision-making, and his own personal transformational journey from obesity to being a normal weight, even slim person, was the inspiration and the basis for the TAKE 5 book.

www.ingramcontent.com/pod-product-compliance
Lightning Source LLC
Chambersburg PA
CBHW060847280326
41934CB00007B/946